EXPOSING THE SPIRITUAL ROOTS OF DISEASE
STUDY GUIDE

DR. HENRY W. WRIGHT

EXPOSING THE SPIRITUAL ROOTS OF DISEASE

STUDY GUIDE

POWERFUL ANSWERS TO YOUR QUESTIONS ABOUT HEALING AND DISEASE PREVENTION

WHITAKER HOUSE

Publisher's Note: This book is not intended to provide medical or psychological advice or to take the place of medical advice and treatment from your personal physician. Those who are having suicidal thoughts or who have been emotionally, physically, or sexually abused should seek help from a mental health professional or qualified counselor. Neither the publisher nor the author nor the author's ministry takes any responsibility for any possible consequences from any action taken by any person reading or following the information in this book. If readers are taking prescription medications, they should consult with their physicians and not take themselves off prescribed medicines without the proper supervision of a physician. Always consult your physician or other qualified healthcare professional before undertaking any change in your physical regimen, whether fasting, diet, medications, or exercise.

All Scripture quotations are taken from the King James Version of the Holy Bible.

EXPOSING THE SPIRITUAL ROOTS OF DISEASE STUDY GUIDE
Powerful Answers to Your Questions About Healing and Disease Prevention

Be in Health®, LLC
4178 Crest Highway
Thomaston, GA 30286
www.beinhealth.com
info@beinhealth.com

ISBN: 979-8-88769-399-6
eBook ISBN: 979-8-88769-400-9
Printed in the United States of America
© 2025 by Be in Health®, LLC. All rights reserved.

Whitaker House
1030 Hunt Valley Circle
New Kensington, PA 15068
www.whitakerhouse.com

Library of Congress Cataloging-in-Publication Data (Pending)

No part of this book may be reproduced or transmitted in any form or by any means, electronic or mechanical—including photocopying, recording, or by any information storage and retrieval system—without permission in writing from the publisher. Please direct your inquiries to permissionseditor@whitakerhouse.com.

1 2 3 4 5 6 7 8 9 10 11 ᰯ 33 32 31 30 29 28 27 26 25

DISCLAIMER

We do not seek to be in conflict with any medical or psychiatric practices, or any church or its religious doctrines, beliefs, or practices. We are not part of medicine or psychology; we are working to make them more effective, believing that many human problems are fundamentally spiritual, with associated physiological and psychological manifestations. This information is intended for your general knowledge only, to give insight into disease, its problems, and possible solutions. It is not a substitute for medical advice or treatment for specific medical conditions or disorders. We do not diagnose or treat disease.

You should seek prompt medical care for any specific health issues. Treatment modalities around your specific health issues are between you and your physician. We are not responsible for a person's disease or their healing. We are administering the Scriptures and what they say about this subject, along with what the medical and scientific communities have observed in line with this insight. There is no guarantee any person will be healed or any disease prevented. The fruits of this teaching will come forth out of the application of the principles and the relationship between each person and God. Be in Health˙ is patterned after 2 Corinthians 5:18–20, 1 Corinthians 12, Ephesians 4, and Mark 16:15–20.

CONTENTS

How to Use This Study Guide 9

Part One: The Foundation for Healing

1. Disease: Happenstance or Planned Event? 13
2. Is Disease a Blessing or a Curse? 21
3. The Biblical Role of Prayer in Healing 29
4. Spirit-Soul-Body Connection 37
5. Pathways of Disease 45

Part Two: Exposing the Roots of Specific Diseases

6. The Spiritual Roots of Allergies 55
7. The Spiritual Roots of Autoimmune Disease 63
8. The Spiritual Roots of Cardiovascular Disease 71
9. The Spiritual Roots of Mental Illness 79
10. The Spiritual Roots of Stress Disorders 87
11. What's Next? 95

What Be in Health Offers 101

About the Author 105

Study Guide Answer Key 107

HOW TO USE THIS STUDY GUIDE

Welcome to *Exposing the Spiritual Roots of Disease Study Guide.* We are excited that you have made the decision to further your understanding of healing and disease prevention according to God's Word. This study guide is designed as supplemental material for *Exposing the Spiritual Roots of Disease* by Dr. Henry W. Wright. This book may be completed independently or may be used in a group setting, such as a Bible study, a Sunday school class, or a prayer group.

Elements of Each Lesson

Chapter Theme

The main idea of each chapter is summarized for emphasis and clarity.

Questions for Reflection

Thought questions are posed as a warmup to lead into the study. (For group study, these questions may be asked before or after reading the Chapter Theme, at the discretion of the leader.)

Exploring Spiritual Roots

Questions and review material are provided to summarize and highlight the principles and truths within each chapter and begin to lead the reader/group participant to personalize what is being studied. Page numbers from the expanded edition of the book *Exposing the Spiritual Roots of Disease* corresponding to the answers to each question are supplied for easy reference. (An answer key for the "Exploring Spiritual Roots" questions may be found beginning on page 107.)

Conclusion

A summary or implication statement is included to put the theme of the chapter into perspective.

Applying Principles of Healing

Thought-provoking questions and suggestions for personal action and prayer are provided to help the individual/group participant apply the study material to their particular life circumstances. This section includes three parts:

1. Thinking It Over
2. Acting on It
3. Praying About It

Testimony

Testimonies are included to give glory to God and encourage the reader to walk in freedom from disease.

PART ONE

THE FOUNDATION FOR HEALING

1

DISEASE: HAPPENSTANCE OR PLANNED EVENT?

Chapter Theme

Some people think that getting a disease is like standing under the wrong tree at the wrong time and getting hit by random, falling fruit. "Why did this happen to me?" they ask. However, the reason for sickness and disease may not be just a random occurrence. Why did it happen to you? Why did you get sick? Some people turn to science and medicine for all their answers. However, as Christians, we need to look closely at what the Word of God says about the spiritual root causes of disease.

Questions for Reflection

1. Have you given any serious consideration to the idea that many chronic diseases may have a spiritual "root cause"?

2. Have you ever considered that living a life perpetually offended and bitter or stressed out can be bad for your body?

3. Did you realize that your spirituality (*spirit*) impacts the way you think (*soul*) and, in turn, impacts the way your *body* functions?

Exploring Spiritual Roots

1. What does the word etiology mean? In medical books, what does the term "unknown etiology" mean? (p. 19)

2. What does the medical community generally offer their patients when facing chronic disease? (p. 19)

3. In contrast, what does the author stand for? (p. 20)

4. What does Father God promise us in Psalm 103:3? (p. 20)

5. As a human being, you are a triune being. You have _____, _____, and you live in _____. (p. 21)

6. What does God want to do in your spirit, soul, and body according to 1 Thessalonians 5:23? (p. 20)

7. What is the root cause of disease? The author believes the root cause of _____ chronic disease is spiritual and is the result of _____. (p. 21)

8. What are the three levels of separation? (p. 21)

9. Therefore, healing begins with _____ to God, yourself, and others. (p. 21)

10. *Separation from the Father*—What are some of the reasons why people feel close to Jesus but separated from Father God? (p. 22)

11. According to 1 John 4:16, what does the Bible tells us about God's love? (p. 22)

12. Many people associate God the Father with _____, and then our heavenly Father is guilty by association. (p. 22)

13. List 3 things that reveal Father God's love for us. (p. 23)

    a. Because of His love for us, God chose _____.

    b. Every good thing that we can think of in life _____.

    c. Because of Jesus's sacrifice on the cross, we have been adopted into God's family. He has given us the privilege to cry out to Him, _____ .

14. To be free and healed, we must _____ God's Word that He truly _____. (p. 23)

15. *Separation from ourselves*—What are some of the ways Satan tempts people to have self-hatred, self-loathing, self-bitterness, and guilt? (p. 24)

16. If we believe we are _____, it is a sure sign that we do not understand the _____ Father God has for us. (p. 24)

17. How do we overcome the lies that Father God doesn't love us? (p, 24)

18. *Separation from others*—What is one of the ways that Satan tempts us to become separated from others? (p. 24)

19. According to Hebrews 12:15, what does bitterness do to us and others around us? (p. 24)

20. If we repent to Father God for bitterness, He will forgive us. Write out the truth of 1 John 1:9. (p. 25)

21. Where did separation in relationships and disease come from? Did they come from God? (p. 25)

22. What is the name Satan translated as? (p. 25)

23. Satan is a great deceiver. What is one of Satan's strongest devices that we see in the temptation of Eve? (p. 27)

24. What happened to Adam and Eve when they sinned? (pp. 27–28)

25. After Adam and Eve sinned, why did God ask Adam, "Who told you?" (p. 28)

26. In contrast, how did Jesus respond when He was tempted by Satan in the wilderness? (p. 28)

27. None of the separation, sin, and disease that mankind has experienced since the garden of Eden

_____. It is all a planned event against us by _____.
(p. 29)

28. After the Fall, a spiritual battle between the kingdom of God and the kingdom of Satan began for the hearts and minds of mankind. Write Ephesians 6:12. (p. 30)

29. Our war is not with other humans. Our war is not even with yourselves. Our war is with an

invisible, evil kingdom ruled by _____, _____, _____,

_____, _____. (p. 30)

30. Our war is with an enemy who wants _____. Becoming bitter, fearful, or disheartened, we will think, speak, and act like Satan and his kingdom—this is

_____. (p. 31)

31. So, what are we to do? We need to receive _____. We need to develop

_____ Scripture. What is the warning in Hosea 4:6 ? (p. 31)

32. To return to correct understanding, we turn _____. What does Psalm 103:2–3 tell us? (pp. 31–32)

33. Perhaps what hinders our faith and our healing from disease is not addressing the stumbling block of sin in our lives before _____. We must be willing to practice the first doctrine of Christ, which is _____, before practicing the second doctrine of Christ, which is _____. (pp. 32–33)

34. What does the Strong's Concordance say is the Greek definition of grace? (p. 33)

35. Is repentance only for unbelievers? (p. 34)

36. List the key roots of many diseases that are elements of Satan's kingdom:

Applying Principles of Healing

Conclusion

For those suffering with chronic disease, the medical and scientific world can only offer "disease management." But Father God wants you to understand the spiritual roots of why we are sick and how you can be set free of disease. It's time to acknowledge that there is an invisible war between the kingdom of God and the kingdom of Satan for our hearts, minds, *and bodies*. It's time to recognize the biblical truth that most disease is not a happenstance, but a planned event by the enemy of our souls. Satan may have his devices or tactics, but God will show you how you can defeat them and be in health. You are meant to be a thriver!

Thinking It Over

1. Have you personally wrestled with believing that Father God loves you and wants the best for your life?

2. Do you believe you will experience what the Word of God promises as you work with Father God to be restored back to proper relationship with Him, yourself, and others?

3. Do you accept what the Bible says are the consequences of sin? *"Know ye not, that to whom ye yield yourselves servants to obey, his servants ye are to whom ye obey; whether of sin unto death, or of obedience unto righteousness?"* (Romans 6:16)

4. Are you willing to travel on this journey to expose the possible spiritual roots of your disease?

Acting on It

1. Read the following Scriptures about the love that Father God has for you. These are the truths of His love: 1 John 3:1; 1 John 4:8,16; Ephesians 2:4–5; Jeremiah 31:3

2. Repent, pray, and ask Father God to forgive you for allowing any of Satan's devices to come between you and Him.

Praying About It

Father God, I want to have knowledge according to Your Word and have correct understanding. Please expose anything in me that has caused me to be separated from You, myself, and others. According to Psalm 139:23–24, "*Search me, O God, and know my heart: try me, and know my thoughts; and see if there by any wicked way in me, and lead me in the way everlasting.*" Thank You that even though Satan has planned evil against me, You want to restore me in relationship with You so that I can walk in wholeness according to Your Word—spirit, soul, and body.

2

IS DISEASE A BLESSING OR A CURSE?

Chapter Theme

Many Christians believe that God is the one who brings disease into their lives. They have been deceived into believing that disease can be a blessing from God to perform something in us. It is vital that we understand the biblical truth that our relationship with and obedience to Father God through Jesus Christ brings us great blessings. It is Satan, the thief, who comes to steal, kill, and destroy what God has created. He comes to reduce or take away the strength of our blessings from God.

Questions for Reflection

1. Have you considered what the blessings and curses Moses warned of in Deuteronomy chapter 28 might look like today?
2. Do you believe there is any way a curse can affect a Christian?
3. How might you have given the devil permission to touch you with a curse?

Exploring Spiritual Roots

1. Near the end of his life, Moses gave the Israelites a warning. What were the clear choices God was offering them between contrasting consequences? According to Deuteronomy 30:19, what had God set before them; what should they choose? (p. 38)

2. Moses reveals the blessings that will *"overtake"* God's people because of their obedience to Him. According to Deuteronomy 28:1–14, list a few of those blessings. (p. 38)

3. However, if God's people chose disobedience instead of blessings, there are many curses that *"shall come upon them and overtake them."* Look up Deuteronomy 28:15–67 and list some of the curses related to disease.

4. *"These blessings shall come on thee, and overtake thee, **if** thou shalt hearken unto the voice of the Lord thy God"* (Deuteronomy 28:2). What is the implication of the Hebrew word "kiy" for the word *if* in this verse? (p. 40)

5. In Deuteronomy 28:15, *"But it shall come to pass, **if** thou wilt not hearken unto the voice of the Lord thy God...curses..."* Moses uses a different Hebrew word "im" for the word *if*. What does it imply this time?

6. Why does the form of the word *"if"* in Deuteronomy 28:15 indicate it *moves slower* than the previous form of *"if"*? (p. 40)

7. Every class of disease known to man is found in the verses of Deuteronomy 28:15–67, and God called them _____. We recognize that these same diseases are plaguing far too many believers today. List some of these diseases. (p. 41)

8. Does God send curses to us? Some people point to Paul's "thorn in the flesh" as coming from God, but there is a problem with this position. What is the problem? (pp. 41–42)

9. If the Bible reveals that disease is evil and a curse, is it possible for God to give us a disease? What does James 1:13 say? (p. 42)

10. Some people are fearful; others are angry, resentful, or bitter. Have you ever wondered why different people have different addictions or weaknesses of character? We have found that it is because

_____. (p. 42)

11. What is a curse? In *Strong's Concordance*, the first word found for the meaning of curse is

_____. The word _____ starts with the

same letters as the word _____. (p. 43)

12. The word "villain" reminds us of John 10:10: *"The thief cometh not, but for to steal, and to kill, and to destroy: I am come that they might have life, and that they might have it more abundantly."* The thief,

_____, is the enemy, the _____, not God! (p. 43)

13. A curse is also the *abatement* of the blessing. What does abatement mean? What does the villain, who is Satan, come to do? (p. 43)

14. Can a Christian be affected by a curse? Proverbs 26:2 tells us that a *"curse causeless shall not come."* What does that mean? (p. 43)

15. According to Galatians 3:13, *"Christ hath redeemed us from the curse of the law."* Didn't Christ's death end the curse brought on mankind by Adam and Eve?

16. However, _____ is how Christians, who are covered by the blood of the Lamb, can be under the burden of a curse from the enemy. (p. 44)

17. A curse that has no cause cannot affect a Christian. But a curse can affect us if

_____.

How do we give the devil this permission? (p. 44)

18. Even though the apostle Paul was a committed follower of Christ, in Romans chapter 7, he confessed that there was a war within him. What two laws were battling for his soul? (p. 45)

19. Paul said in Romans 7:22–23, "*For I delight in the law of God after the inward man: but I see*

_____ , *warring against the law of my mind, and*

_____." This battle of the law of sin against the

law of God that happened within Paul _____. (pp. 44–45)

20. When Paul talks about the law of God, he is referring to God's nature. List some of the attributes of God that reflect His righteousness. (p. 45)

21. On the other side of the war, the nature of Satan is found under the category of the law of sin. List some of the evil characteristics of Satan's nature. (p. 45)

22. In 2 Timothy 2:24–26, Paul says that the servant of the Lord can be ensnared and taken captive by whom? (p. 48)

23. Jesus linked the law of sin _____ more than once in the New Testament. After Jesus healed the paralyzed man lying beside the pool of Bethesda, what did he say to him? (pp. 48–49)

24. When healing someone, Jesus often used the phrases _____ and _____ together. By joining them together, what is He indicating? (p. 49)

25. We shouldn't be discouraged about the battle we face between the law of sin and the law of God. Jesus's life, death, and resurrection brought us the Father's grace and mercy. What is the Strong's definition of grace? (p. 50)

26. Grace's companion is mercy. What is mercy defined as according to Strong's? (p. 50)

27. If we find sin in our hearts, how may we now respond to God because we love Him and want to live in Him? (p. 50)

Applying Principles of Healing

Conclusion

So, is disease a blessing or a curse? There are two laws battling inside you: the law of God and the law of sin. The question for you to consider is this: Which law are you being influenced by today? The plain truth is that Satan's kingdom wants you to believe God is responsible for sin and responsible for your illness. If Satan can keep you confused about the source of sickness and convince you that there are no curses or consequences for sin, you can never be free. The simple fact is this: there are sicknesses that are the result of our accepting the law of sin into our lives. God desires to set us free from the law of sin through the power of Jesus Christ. It is important to settle our hearts that indeed only *good* gifts come from the Father of lights—Father God.

Thinking It Over

1. When you practice the law of sin after you know the law of God, you are calling God's Word evil and Satan's word good. In what ways do you recognize that you have done this in your own life? Are there any areas where you have not made God the Lord of your life, and you have given Satan a legal right to your life?

2. How do you see God's grace and mercy working in your life?

3. Do you relate to Paul's struggle by finding that sometimes the harder you try, the more behind you get?

4. Through Jesus's sacrifice at the cross, the devil was defeated. And by the power of the Holy Spirit, we have a Comforter who resides with us. What do you think this daily journey should look like for believers as we learn to overcome Satan's kingdom day by day?

Acting On It

1. Read Deuteronomy chapters 28 and 30 carefully to understand God's warning to His people about the consequences of obedience versus disobedience.

2. Reread Romans chapter 7 about the apostle Paul's battle within between the law of God and the law of sin.

Praying About It

Father God, thank You that You don't tempt us with evil but have provided a way for us to recover ourselves from the snare of the devil. I don't want to live in disobedience over anything that was paid for by Jesus's obedience to You. I choose to make Jesus the Lord of my life in every area so that the devil has no right to my life and my generations. I want to have blessings overtake me according to Your Word. Thank You that Your truth restores me and makes me free.

Healing Testimony

A Journey of Freedom

My primary diagnoses were hypothyroidism, ovarian cysts, endometriosis, chronic urinary tract infections, chronic strep throat infections, ulcers, irritable bowel syndrome, eczema, infertility, major depression, dysmenorrhea, asthma, anxiety with panic attacks, and candida.

In my desperation, I began seeking alternative medical treatments, participating in yoga, utilizing magnets and muscle testing for healing, and shopping only at health food stores. I was trying to control food and supplements because my life was so out of control. My allergies had become unmanageable, and I was reacting negatively to many different things in my environment. I had become allergic to perfume, laundry soap, all molds, candles, polyester clothing, smoke, EMF frequencies from smart meters and cell phones, bleach, cats, space heaters, and ink from copiers. I had visited the ER multiple times for breathing problems.

In 2017, I hit bottom as I became homebound due to all my allergies. A friend told me that I needed to read the book *A More Excellent Way*. As I read it, the healing began, and all the Scripture just washed over my soul. From that point on, I had hope.

God's timing is perfect. A month later, I signed up online for a free Be In Health webinar called Overcoming Allergies. During that livestream, I learned that a broken heart could lead to fear and a compromised immune system. Dr. Henry W. Wright began to talk about the connection between lack of love and fear. I was so hungry for the truth. He talked about how important it is to meditate on what God says about you by reading Psalm 139. He suggested that reading this psalm every night before bed for a year was better than any prescription drug you could take. I decided to follow his advice, and for a year I read it and studied how God created me fearfully and wonderfully. I focused on verse 10, which says, *"Even there shall thy hand lead me, and thy right hand shall hold me."* For the first time, I received help from someone without guilt or shame.

I was so excited, so I enrolled in For My Life Online. After watching the teaching on bitterness, I realized that I had been bitter against my mother for her absence in my life and bitter against God for my years of sickness. I cried and repented to the Father for my wrong attitude. As the poison of bitterness came out through my repentance, my health began to improve dramatically. I began to venture out of the house, visiting the grocery store and going out to restaurants with my husband and son. My body started to feel more relaxed and at ease. I was beginning to walk in peace with my heavenly Father.

In the summer of 2019, our family went to Georgia to participate in the For My Life Retreat in person. I had not traveled in several years due to my illnesses, but Father God was with us the whole way. Shortly before going, I was reading Psalm 142:7, which says, *"Bring my soul out of prison, that I may praise thy name: the righteous shall compass me about; for thou shalt deal bountifully with me."* I wrote this on a note and attached it to my bathroom mirror. Through the staff at Be in Health, I saw how God began to fulfill that Scripture. My marriage was still in a rocky place, and that week there was repentance and healing.

My six-year journey has been a highway, where I have learned to walk more in *His* ways and less in my own. Today, I have so much to be thankful for: healing from allergies, my marriage has been restored, and my son no longer experiences allergies, chronic migraine headaches, and nightmares that he was having due to the stress in our family. Many broken relationships have been restored as Father God has directed me to repent and humble myself before Him.

—Kathy

3

THE BIBLICAL ROLE OF PRAYER IN HEALING

Chapter Theme

Our God is a healing God. It is important to search the Scriptures for any direction He gives us concerning healing. In James 5:14–15, we read, *"Is any sick among you? let him call for the elders of the church; and let them pray over him, anointing him with oil in the name of the Lord: and the prayer of faith shall save the sick, and the Lord shall raise him up…"* Laying hands on and praying for people to be healed is in God's Word. We do the same. However, consider the rest of this verse in James. It says, *"…and if he have committed sins, they shall be forgiven him."* It is vital to look at the role that sin and forgiveness have in the healing of God's people.

Questions for Reflection

1. Have you considered whether prayer is the only plan that God gives us for the healing of disease?
2. Is it possible the church is only addressing part of the problem when they pray for healing?
3. Do you need a change in spirituality to come back to peace? Are there any lies you have believed that you need to repent for believing?

Exploring Spiritual Roots

1. What is the main action listed in James 5:14–15 that produces healing from sickness? What other step to healing occurs in James 5:15? (p. 54)

2. Many Christians do not want to believe they need to repent. They think the word *repent* is only used _____. What is the truth from Romans 3:23? (p. 54)

3. Medical research revealed years ago that forgiveness and unforgiveness affect human health. What does the Bible call unforgiveness? _____ People want to be healed without doing what? (p. 55)

4. In the example of the woman with stage IV breast cancer, why didn't the author want to pray for her? Write the Scripture verse from 1 John 5:17. (p. 56)

5. What did the author mean when he said it was a sin *unto death?* (p. 56)

6. Unforgiveness is unrighteousness; therefore, what law are you following if you follow unforgiveness? (p. 57)

7. After the woman with breast cancer admitted she had bitterness, what did she do? (pp. 57–58)

8. What does Matthew 6:15 say? (pp. 57–58)

9. How did healing occur for the woman with breast cancer? What does James 1:22 tell us? (p. 59)

10. Repentance is not a bad word. Having to repent doesn't mean that

_____. Paul was speaking to

_____ when he talked about repentance in 2 Timothy 2:26. (p. 59)

11. What does the author believe are two things we need to do to be successful in our relationships with God and others? (p. 59)

12. We experience repentance from our sins when we first turn to God to acknowledge Jesus Christ's death and resurrection on our behalf. That is _____. We need to allow God to continually change us. That is _____. (p. 60)

13. What is sanctification? (p. 60)

14. It's important that we don't react to God's truth about sin in our life by

_____. Why does the Holy Spirit convict us of sin? (p. 61)

15. God reveals sanctification to us in His Word. According to 2 Corinthians 3:18,

_____. In what tense are the words *we are changed into the same image?* What does that mean? (p. 61)

16. 1 Thessalonians 5:23 states, *"The very God of peace sanctify you wholly; and I pray God your whole spirit and soul and body be preserved blameless unto the coming of our Lord Jesus Christ."* Jesus hasn't returned yet, so what must we remember? (p. 61)

17. According to Romans 12:2, what should we allow to happen to our minds? (p. 61)

18. We are saved by God's forgiveness and mercy, but what must we walk out on a daily basis? (p. 62)

19. We must make a quality decision to do what? (p. 62)

20. What happens when we have a proper relationship with Father God by praying, reading the Bible, and applying His instructions? This is an essential fruit _____. (p. 63)

21. What happens when we do the opposite and listen to Satan's kingdom instead? (p. 63)

22. The sin of bitterness is one major area where we can become a reflection of Satan's kingdom. When we are wronged by someone, what two opposing decisions do we face? (p. 63)

23. How do the degrees of bitterness worsen once the root of unforgiveness has taken hold? (p. 64)

24. If we choose to hold a record of wrongs against another person, what will it likely do? (p. 64)

25. List two major insights Be in Health has gained from our experience with the spiritual roots of breast cancer. (pp. 64–65)

26. List at least 5 characteristics from the cancer profile found on page 67.

27. The overarching thread that ties together the experiences and tendencies on this list is

_____. When someone is unable to address

conflict or disappointment without _____; they might

_____. (p.68)

28. Even if we lose everything we have, we must be willing to

_____. Our hope cannot be based upon

_____. (p. 69)

Applying Principles of Healing

Conclusion

Prayer has a scriptural place in healing, but repentance and sanctification play an important role in disease prevention and becoming free from disease. According to James 5:14–15, we can anoint the sick with oil *"in the name of the Lord: and the prayer of faith shall save the sick."* Yet, the verse goes on to say, *"and if he have committed sins, they shall be forgiven him."*

You can do a lot to prevent disease in your life when you communicate openly with Father God, admit when you have fallen into sin, repent of the sin, ask His forgiveness, choose not to follow after that sin in the future, and allow Him to transform you into His image. God is not going to live your life for you! You must take ownership in this victory. It's time to be transparent when you have missed the mark. That is God's plan for you. As a result, your body will rejoice and be in health!

Thinking It Over

1. When people see you, do they see a "non-bitter" person? Or do they see a *loving* person? You can choose to love.
2. How do you live out the command to forgive your enemies? Can you release every person and their sins against you to Father God, and relinquish control to Father God to be your defender? (pp. 66–67)
3. What idols of expectations and hope might you have in your life instead of your ultimate hope being in the Lord? Has this led to any hope deferred in your life?

Acting on It

1. Ask the Father to show you whose sins you might have taken into your body through the sin of holding a record of wrongs against another person. Ask Him for forgiveness for agreeing with a spirit of bitterness toward any person who has hurt you.

2. Ask the Father if there is anyone you might need to repent to. Ask the Father to forgive you for any wrong expectations or hope.

3. Entrust your life *with* Him and release your hopes *to* Him. He is your ultimate hope.

Praying About It

Father, I want to live out Your command to forgive my enemies. I do not call sin "okay." It is evil. Help me to decide to release each person and their sin against me to You. I want to engage with You and have You teach me how to love in a world that may not love me. Please show me how to forgive and re-engage even with those people who may have done harm to me in the past. And if this is not possible, help me to love them and pray for the restoration of relationship even at a distance. I want my prayer life with You to focus on being part of the spiritual solution instead of the spiritual pollution of sin. Help me to be transformed into Your image so that I might display Your nature.

Healing Testimony

Healed From Thyroid Cancer

I was diagnosed with thyroid cancer with lymph node involvement. Friends told me about Be in Health, so I bought quite a few of their books. Eventually, I was able to go to the For My Life Retreat in Thomaston, Georgia. There, the Bible teachings I had learned over the years suddenly came together and made sense. Though I did not fully understand it yet, it was the beginning of letting go, trusting God, and believing His Word is true.

During the teachings, I received an understanding of God's perfect love for the first time and an enlightenment of what fear is and how it works—recognizing where I had allowed fear to hijack me from a relationship with God and from a satisfying life. I recognized the bitterness in my heart toward others, and why forgiving them and letting go of the offenses was the only way God could get to my heart and bring the healing and restitution that I did not even know I wanted. Once I was able to forgive, it snowballed into wholeheartedly believing God loves me and that I can trust my heart is safe with Him.

After attending a few retreats at Be in Health, I had my yearly exam for the thyroid cancer. The tests came back looking suspicious, so I needed to have a few additional procedures done. I really had to grapple with some things during that time. The temptations to go into fear, isolation, despair—even thoughts of suicide—were continuously bombarding my mind. During one of the procedures, I was angry, thinking God "knew what was going to happen" and asking, "Why is He making me go through this again?" Even in fear and anger, I heard Him ask, "So this is My fault? Are you accusing Me of giving you cancer?" Then I heard (not audibly, just inside my head), "I come to give life abundant; the devil brings death and destruction." I repented and asked forgiveness for accusing God. The choice to believe and flip the thought was weird and unfamiliar, but I knew it was a pivotal moment in how I see God and how I choose to think and believe. Not just about my health, but about trusting that He wants good for me, that I am worthy of good things. The reports from my tests came back clear! The night I got the news, I asked the Lord what I should read in the Bible and heard Psalm 30. Psalm 30:2 says, "O Lord my God, I cried to You, and *You have healed me.*" The moment I read that, I knew God has taken away the cancer, and I am healed!

—Melissa

4

SPIRIT-SOUL-BODY CONNECTION

Chapter Theme

The spirit-soul-body connection provides us with the understanding of how God speaks to us and influences us to follow after His nature and His Word. It also exposes how Satan speaks to us in our thoughts in an attempt to influence us toward his evil nature. We need to understand how God and Satan both speak to us in order to understand fully the spiritual roots of disease. This is why we look at the role our mind plays in disease—this is the spirit-soul(mind)-body connection.

Questions for Reflection

1. Have you ever considered that there might be a connection between your spirit, your soul, and your body related to your health?
2. Have you ever wondered how the enemy could possibly deposit a thought into your mind?
3. Is it possible that your thoughts, or what you dwell upon, might be making you sick?

Exploring Spiritual Roots

1. Where do our thoughts come from? (p. 73)

2. Who can and cannot have the mind of Christ? (pp. 73–74)

3. How do we acquire the mind of Christ? (p. 74)

4. We know that the Holy Spirit of God is a Spirit. Satan is a spirit. We are each a
   _____. Our body interacts with the physical world, but
   _____. (p. 74)

5. God communicates with us Spirit to spirit. Unfortunately, _____ also
   communicates with us spirit to spirit. We receive thoughts at the _____ and record
   them at the _____. Thoughts from the enemy can
   _____. (p. 74)

6. Why do we think negative or evil thoughts are our own thoughts? (p. 75)

7. Give examples of the kinds of thoughts Satan might repeat in our minds. (p. 75)

8. What happens if we embrace the enemy's thoughts and take ownership of them? What does the
   Bible call these thoughts? (p. 75)

9. We all have brainwaves as part of our cognition. Because of the spirit-soul-body connection, there
   are three specific brain waves that the author relates to his scriptural understanding of how human
   beings function. What are they?

10. What are beta brainwaves responsible for? What do the beta waves form a connection between? (p. 76)

11. What are alpha brainwaves a part of? What do alpha waves form a connection with? (p. 76)

12. What do theta waves form a junction between? Theta brainwaves are how both

    _____. (p. 76)

13. God wants to influence us from within by His Spirit and by His Word. He uses

    _____ to speak to us from within, to train us in

    _____. The kingdom of darkness wants to influence us from within as

    well; the enemy _____. (p. 76)

14. We will never get to the spiritual root of disease if we don't understand

    _____. (p. 76)

15. How does your short-term memory become integrated permanently into your brain cells as long-term memory? (p. 77)

16. Those long-term memories and images, _____, now become

    _____. What three things are affected? (p. 77)

17. Satan will train us through long-term memory with _____.
However, God will train us through long-term memory as we

_____. (p. 77)

18. What happens when we embrace the temptations and thoughts of the enemy instead of embracing the truth of God's Word? Did Jesus cast out people's emotions in the Gospels? (p. 77)

19. People are afraid that the word _____ means being _____ by devils.

Christians _____ be owned by devils. What are two alternate translations for the word *possessed?* (p. 78)

20. How do we know that evil spirits exist? Because the Word tells us so. Write out 2 Timothy 1:7. (p. 78)

21. Some Christians claim that evil spirits _____, and that the term *flesh* that Paul uses several times is essentially our _____ that is leading us into sin as if by instinct. (p. 80)

22. Through the spirit-soul-body connection, it is not the physical body that makes us sin, but

_____. We make decisions in our soul that

produce _____. (pp. 80–81)

23. The author's position is that although we sin, we _____. This key teaching, known as _____, helps us understand the spirit-soul-body connection because it addresses evil spirits as being _____. (p. 81)

24. What is the primary way that Satan's kingdom brings condemnation and confusion into the lives of Christians? If we believe that evil thoughts and feelings originate with us, what are we stuck with? (p. 81)

25. How can we be separated from these evil thoughts and evil spirits? (p. 81)

26. Once we are set free, we can begin a new journey to do what? (p. 81)

27. Is temptation a sin? It only becomes sin when we embrace _____. Don't feel condemned. We don't _____! (p. 84)

28. At Be in Health, we teach what we call the 8 Rs to Freedom to make you free! (pp. 85–86)

   Recognize. _____

   Responsibility. _____

   Repent. _____

   Renounce. _____

   Remove it. _____

Resist. _____

Rejoice. _____

Restore. _____

29. Once we are free, what should we do with the thoughts that Satan tries to bring to our mind according to 2 Corinthians 10:5? (p. 87) We can choose to follow the Word of God

_____.

Applying Principles of Healing

Conclusion

The spirit-soul-body connection opens our eyes to the truth that there is a way for God to speak His nature and thoughts into our minds, and a way for the enemy to plant thoughts into our minds as well. Embracing the enemy's thoughts instead of God's Word leads us to sin. The point is that the core of our struggle against sin is not with ourselves but with an evil kingdom determined to destroy our lives. Through the spirit-soul-body connection, Satan is determined to make us believe that we are evil, and that sin is an integral part of us.

This is how he does it: A spirit of bitterness wants you to believe you are *a bitter person* and that it is a part of your original thought process. A spirit of fear will make you feel afraid and lead you to the conclusion that you are just *a fearful person*. These evil spirits want you to believe that they are *you*! They are not! God desires for you to see that even if we sin, *you are not your sin*! You can be separated from the enemy to live in health and freedom!

Thinking It Over

1. Why do many Christians refuse to address the existence of evil spirits? After studying this chapter, what do you believe?

2. The Word clearly tells us that the spirit of fear exists. What can an evil spirit do to us if we give it permission and dwell on it?

3. What startling statement does Paul make in Romans 7:17? Who or what commits the things Paul does not want to do?

Acting on It

1. Put into practice the first 5 Rs with a specific sin you have recognized in your life. Recognize it, take responsibility for agreeing with it, repent to God for participating with it, renounce it from your life, and remove the law of sin from you.

2. If the temptation to sin in that area comes back after you are free, take that thought captive by casting it down in the name of Jesus. This is the 6th R.

3. Do the 7th and 8th R's: give God glory for your freedom! And be ready to help restore others with the same freedom you have received.

Praying About It

Father God, thank You that You don't tempt us with evil but instead have provided a way for us to recover ourselves from the snare of the devil. I don't want to live in disobedience over anything that was paid for by Jesus's obedience to You. I make Jesus the Lord of my life in every area so that the devil has no right to my life and my generations. I want to have blessings overtake me according to Your Word. Thank You that Your truth restores me and makes me free.

Healing Testimony

Our God Can Do Anything!

Prior to being introduced to Be in Health, I was leading a very structured, health-issue-focused life working to maximize my energy so I could function. Unfortunately, the various therapies and diets—along with my low energy—were isolating me. They also consumed a lot of time, money, and thought. It was a very "me-focused" lifestyle with lots of doctors' appointments and therapies. I had food sensitivities, fall and spring allergies, multiple chemical sensitivities (MCS), irritable bowel syndrome (IBS), mild adrenal insufficiency (which gives symptoms that are far from mild), chronic Lyme disease, and hypoglycemia. I needed lots of sleep to function and days of recovery if I had a long day. I took my own food with me everywhere I went because I was on a gluten-free, very low-sugar, dairy-free, sorghum-flour-free, low-fodmap diet to function.

One day, a pastor shared with me that his wife had been healed after attending a For My Life Retreat, so I began listening to Be in Health YouTube testimonies and teachings focused on allergies. After determining that Be in Health was a solid Christian ministry, I signed up for the For My Life online class. Once I finished the class, I was able to eat dairy products successfully for the first time in more than ten years. I now had hope!

I decided to go to the Walk Out Workshop (WOW) in Thomaston, Georgia, because I knew there was much more I needed to learn. I knew God was calling me to go but traveling alone was a big challenge because of my concerns of becoming incapacitated by a chemical allergic reaction that would make it impossible for me to think clearly. My friends and family declined my offer to come along, so I determined I would go on my own. I knew God was calling me to go to the WOW Retreat, and I knew that when God calls you, He equips you. I decided to fly to Atlanta and rent a car. I was a little intimidated, but I made it!

On the first day of the Walk Out Workshop, I found a missing piece of my healing: the 8 Rs. I hadn't realized how to implement that tool in my life. During that week, I learned how to fight fear. I grew in my understanding of my authority in Christ. I understood that God's voice is *never* condemning. It may be convicting, but *not* condemning. I learned more about how to fight the enemy's attacks. I left the workshop experiencing great freedom and great peace.

I have been healed of inhalant allergies, multiple chemical sensitivities (MCS), mold allergies, asthma, chronic fatigue syndrome (CFS), food sensitivities, hypoglycemia, IBS, persistent leg cramps, mild adrenal insufficiency, and chronic Lyme. I have had five thyroid blood lab tests and have had thyroid prescriptions reduced from two to one. Even more than the physical healing, the peace that I now have is incredible! I know that our God can do anything!

—Myra

5

PATHWAYS OF DISEASE

Chapter Theme

Now that we understand how our thoughts can be influenced by God or by the enemy, it's time to study the connection between thought and physiology. We need to understand how our bodies are constructed—and how God's plan can be thwarted by the decisions we make in our thought life. If we have a long-term memory full of thoughts that oppose God's Word, our body systems will malfunction because they are without peace or without *ease*. This chapter exposes the specific biological pathways that Satan uses to bring *dis-ease*.

Questions for Reflection

1. Have you ever considered that by agreeing with a spirit of fear's thoughts in your mind, something could misfire in your body, causing all types of problems for your health?

2. Can examining God's creative miracle of your body and what medical science can see happening in disease provide clues to the spiritual roots of disease?

3. Could understanding how the spiritual roots of disease work give you the opportunity to keep your body in homeostasis and to keep disease far away from you?

Exploring Spiritual Roots

1. List the three amazing foundational blocks for human development formed in the earliest days after conception. (p. 93)

2. Which body systems are developed from the ectoderm? (p. 93)

3. In Chart 2, what does the author see as Satan's main device that attacks the systems from the ectoderm? And what does the author list as God's solution? (p. 93)

4. Which systems are developed from the mesoderm? (p. 93)

5. In Chart 2, what does the author see as Satan's main device that attacks the systems from the mesoderm? What does the author list as God's solution? (p. 93)

6. Which systems are developed from the endoderm? (p. 93)

7. In Chart 2, what does the author see as Satan's main device that attacks the systems from the endoderm? What does the author list as God's solution? (p. 93)

8. All of these systems are highly responsive and regulated by a flow that originates from which body part? (p. 93)

9. What part of our nervous system gives us the control over our bodily movements? In contrast, what was our involuntary or sympathetic nervous system created to do? Give examples of body systems that work involuntarily. (p. 94)

10. What does the author mean by dis-ease of function? (p. 94)

11. What is the author's definition of dis-ease? Dis-ease is exactly what it sounds like:

    _____. (p. 94)

12. What does the limbic system of the brain regulate? To understand the roots of disease, which glands in the brain should we focus on? (p. 94)

13. The amygdalae glands are responsible for what we call _____ to emergency situations, stress, and fear. They play a vital role in

    _____. What else are the amygdalae involved in? (p. 94)

14. What pea-sized gland in the brain is vitally important for understanding the spiritual roots of disease? This tiny gland is the pathway to both _____. (p. 95)

15. The endocrine system is a chemical messenger system that includes which three important glands? What is the primary purpose of these glands? (p. 95)

16. Which of these glands is considered the control center of the entire endocrine system? (p. 95)

17. The main role of the hypothalamus is to keep our body in homeostasis. What does homeostasis mean? What happens when it isn't maintained? (p. 96)

18. As the control center, the hypothalamus regulates numerous bodily activities. List several of them. (p. 96)

19. What happens when the hypothalamus is not functioning normally? (p. 97)

20. The hypothalamus gland plays a central role in the spirit-soul-body connection. It is how we process _____. Most important for this study is _____. (p. 97)

21. What happens when we meditate on or replay thoughts of fear, anxiety, bitterness, anger, or self-hatred? (p. 97)

22. What occurs next in the limbic system? (p. 97)

23. What happens when the hypothalamus receives these negative messages? (p. 97)

24. What have these overwhelming thoughts and the evil spirit behind them done to the hypothalamus? What can living in this way lead to over time? (p. 97)

25. In Chart 5, we can see the lengthy list of diseases that result from a lack of homeostasis or disfunction in the hypothalamus gland. List some of them. (pp. 97–98)

26. How does the enemy use the hypothalamus? How is our spirit-man involved in this connection between the mind, the hypothalamus gland, and disease? (p. 99)

27. How do our soul and body come into homeostasis? In contrast, what happens when the devil is successful with temptation in our thought life? (p. 99)

28. Explain the three steps in the pathway to disease:

   a. The enemy tempts us with thoughts that are part of the law of sin and that oppose the Word of God, such as _____.

   b. If we embrace those unrighteous thoughts and meditate or dwell on them instead of on the Word of God, _____.

   c. These elevated negative emotions, and the spirits behind them, are then communicated _____. Over time, what happens if we live this way? (pp. 99–100)

29. What is the only gland that Satan and his kingdom need to move us in the direction of dis-ease? Instead of our body functioning as God intended, what do we end up with? (p. 100)

Applying Principles of Healing

Conclusion

God has created us to be in health. He has created our bodies to function in homeostasis or in balance. Unfortunately, Satan understands how the human body functions. As we have seen, all he needs is one small gland to set this whole mess in motion. The enemy understands what he needs to do to send the hypothalamus into imbalance and to wreak havoc with our health. He is good at it—but God is so much bigger. He will give us victory over the enemy's plan! That is why we have shared the knowledge of this battle so you will know how to fight Satan's plan of disease for your life. Do not dwell on the enemy's evil temptations! Instead, meditate on the powerful truth in God's Word!

Thinking It Over

1. What is the connection between the soul and the body? How can improper spirituality impact your body systems?

2. Did you realize that medical science can see the connection between anxiety (fear) and heart palpitations, hostility and artery thrombosis, and shame and irritable bowel syndrome? What other connections that we have discussed might be made as medical science progresses?

3. The flight-or-fight response is meant to be a short-term plan for emergency situations only. What might the physical effects be upon someone who has been in a constant state of fight-or-flight for a long period of time?

Acting on It

1. Repent for dwelling on the enemy's thoughts; dwell on God's thoughts instead.

2. Make a list of ten Scriptures that remind you of God's thoughts and promises toward you.

3. Decide to dwell on and follow the Word of God despite how you might feel.

Praying Over It

Father, thank You that Your Word is true and provides a solution for every situation I am facing. I speak peace to my amygdala and hypothalamus in the name of Jesus that they may come into homeostasis as God intends and cause all my body systems to come into proper alignment. Father, thank You for knowledge so that I can know how to fight Satan's plan of disease for my life and my generations. You are so much bigger than the enemy. Help me to meditate on the truth from Your Word so that it becomes part of my long-term memory and my physiology. Thank You for creating my body to prosper and be in health even as my soul prospers.

Healing Testimony

Taking My Life Back

In 2021, I started experiencing a vibrating feeling in my back, which only stopped when all the electronics around me were turned off. The vibrating feeling would come back whenever lights, ceiling fans, phones, Wi-Fi, or the TV were on in the house. I would feel lightheaded, nauseous, and in pain. My family suffered greatly because of this. Nobody could turn on electronics, and I was completely isolated in the dark, being unable to leave my bedroom. I felt like I was dying; my skin and lips were pale gray, and I had suicidal thoughts. I couldn't even wear my clothes because our washer had mold. I could barely wear anything, or I would start shaking uncontrollably. Even the faucets began to make me sick. I could no longer bathe or wash my hands in the water without feeling ill. One night, my symptoms were so bad that I felt like my nasal passages and throat were closing.

Thankfully, a dear woman from our church sent me the book *A More Excellent Way* by Dr. Henry W. Wright, which was filled with Scripture and unbelievable, life-changing knowledge. As I read the book, God began to do a work in me! I had been consumed by fear for most of my life, as well as panic, anxiety, and stress. I repented, and God gave me His peace and began to teach me what His Word of truth said. I attended a For My Life Retreat, and my healing came quickly once I learned that every symptom I had been dealing with was a lie from Satan's kingdom.

My ability to take my life back and be healed by God has *only* resulted from a lot of repentance and deep spiritual work with the Lord! I still have symptoms that try to come back, but I now know they are lies. I cast them down in Jesus's name, or I just tell those familiar spirits out loud that they no longer have access to me, and I am God's child. I speak Scripture out loud, and they must submit to the Word of God and leave me alone!

Now I can go to restaurants, I have returned to church, and I have access to my entire house again. Every day feels like I am living a new day. I thought my life was over, but now it feels like it has just begun! I was a captive, but God loved me so much that He gave me the knowledge I needed to be released from Satan's snare. And now He is using me to set others free and to lay hands on people for healing. Praise be to the Lord God Almighty!

—Michelle

PART TWO

EXPOSING THE ROOTS OF SPECIFIC DISEASES

6

THE SPIRITUAL ROOTS OF ALLERGIES

Chapter Theme

Allergies are defined as "an abnormal reaction by the immune system to a substance that is usually not harmful." Having allergies means we are allergic to God's creation, things He meant for us to enjoy. That is not God's plan. Doctors and researchers aren't sure why some people get allergies, and they do not believe allergies can be cured, only managed by medication and lifestyle changes. In other words, allergies have an "unknown etiology." However, the common spiritual root to allergies is fear. Fear often is produced by a broken heart and does not allow people to give or receive love in relationships. However, God loves us, and He intends for each of us to be free of allergies!

Questions for Reflection

1. Have you ever been fearful? Have you ever seen a fearful person?
2. Have you ever observed the facial expressions and body language of someone who is really stressed out? What does it look and feel like?
3. What do you think causes stress? Is it possible that stress is the result of being afraid? Could stress and fear be synonymous?

Exploring Spiritual Roots

1. When we are stressed out, we are not at _____. According to 1 John 4:18, what does fear bring? (p. 104)

2. Identify the spiritual defect behind "stress." How does an evil spirit manifest in us? (p. 104)

3. How have several modern Bible translations changed the wording of 2 Timothy 1:7? Who calls it a spirit of fear? What problem does this cause? (p. 104)

4. Hebrews 11:1 is a strong statement about faith: *"Now faith is the substance of things hoped for, the evidence of things not seen"* On the opposite side of faith, fear is

_____! While faith is greater than fear, in what two ways are they equal? (p. 105)

5. Jesus said, *"According to your faith be it unto you"* (Matthew 9:29). How does the enemy want to replace that verse? (p. 105)

6. What are allergies a result of? (p. 105)

7. The primary spiritual cause of allergies is _____

_____. The result is additional _____ in all relationships. What does this fear cause us to do? (p. 106)

8. _____ is a naturally occurring steroid released by the adrenal glands. It has its function, especially _____, that could be dangerous. (p. 106)

9. What is a "cortisol drip?" If we continue to manifest anxiety and stress in our life, what will the drip, drip of cortisol do? (p. 106)

10. Does cortisol destroy the immune system because of a lack of nutrition? (p. 106)

11. Are we really allergic to anything or are we experiencing a biological phenomenon of fear and the consequences of cortisol release? (p. 106)

12. What did God create the human immune system to accomplish? (p. 106)

13. What is the function of our T cells and B cells? (p. 107)

14. Both healthy cells and invader cells, such as bacteria and viruses, have a marker called _____. When things function the way God created them to, the T cells and B cells recognize _____. (p. 108)

15. What happens with excessive cortisol in our body? The T cells _____. The B cells mistakenly create antibodies _____ _____. (p. 108)

16. When our immune system is malfunctioning, and the B cells attack natural substances, what will our body overproduce? What are the symptoms of this overproduction? (p. 108)

17. What does the medical community give us to try to build up our immune system against allergies? Why isn't this the answer? What do doctors prescribe for the overabundance of histamine in our body that produced the allergic "reactions"? (p. 109)

18. How do we keep our immune system healthy according to the Word of God? God's nature includes the nine fruit of the Spirit. To have a healthy immune system, our nature should reflect God's nature in Galatians 5:22–23. Write the verses below. (p. 109)

19. In the example of the baby boy who had severe eczema on his face, how was the baby healed of his disease? (p. 110)

20. In the example of the toddler girl who developed seasonal allergies, what did her parents discover? (pp. 111–112)

21. When the author prayed for wisdom on how to minister to the woman with MCS/EI, God led him to Proverbs 17:22: *"A merry heart doeth good like a medicine: but a broken spirit drieth the bones."* It was a revelation that _____

_____. (p. 113)

22. This woman with MCS/EI was healed in a matter of days. What steps had she taken for her healing? (pp. 113–114)

23. If we have a broken heart, we have been *pierced*. What does being pierced mean? What does the enemy use these tragedies to do to us? (p. 114)

24. How does the piercing become a *wound* that will not heal? What should we do instead? (pp. 114–115)

25. How can we break away from the patterns of sin and desolation in ourselves and our family tree? (p. 115)

26. A broken heart does not allow people to _____. They also believe that no one understands _____. (p. 115)

27. The common spiritual root of multiple and simple allergies is _____. Freedom and healing come from repenting of agreeing with these tormenting thoughts of fear and embracing

    _____. (p. 116)

28. When we choose to dwell on and follow the Word of God despite what we feel, with time,

    _____. (p. 117)

29. Even when the enemy comes back to remind us of certain thoughts or issues that make us afraid, we shouldn't shrink back. We must go to _____

    _____. (p. 117)

Applying Principles of Healing

Conclusion

For the sake of your health, get rid of as much fear as you can because God is not giving it to you; the enemy is. Don't let fear and anxiety lead you into disease. Psalm 34:4 says, *"I sought the Lord, and he heard me, and delivered me from all my fears."* Let the Holy Spirit form His incredible nature in you. The enemy might still tempt you, but he cannot touch you. Take ownership of your life! With time, our bodies will stop responding to the training of fear. Those who have been healed have observed their bodies no longer reacting to fear. The hypersensitivity and inflammation associated with allergies were healed. Their immune systems were healed, and their hearts were made whole. There is hope. If you seek the Lord and call upon His name, you will be delivered. That's a promise you need to embrace!

Thinking It Over

1. Are you surprised to learn that you (and/or others) are not really allergic to anything?
2. What are the keys to defeating allergies?
3. Like the woman with MCS/EI, if you were asked the following questions, what would your response be: Who damaged you? Who was supposed to love you but didn't? Who broke your heart?

Acting on It

1. If there was anyone who broke your heart, take some time to repent to God for taking on any bitterness toward them. Then take some time to forgive the person or persons who may have hurt you.
2. According to 1 John 4:18, perfect love casts out fear. Spend time thanking God for His perfect love, receive it, and then choose to believe it. Search the Word and write down 10 verses about God's love for you.
3. Ask God if there are any ways that you have isolated yourself from others out of distrust or fear of being hurt. Are there ways for you to come into fellowship with others and begin to trust again?
4. If applicable, repent to God for not accepting yourself or agreeing with guilt and shame. Ask God to help you accept and love yourself; remember, you are not the problem!

Praying About It

Father God, thank You that Your perfect love casts out fear. Thank You that You have not given me a spirit of fear, but a spirit of power, love, and a sound mind. Thank You for making me accepted in the Beloved, and for choosing me in You before the foundation of the world. Thank You that when I seek You, You hear me and deliver me from all of my fears. I receive Your love for me, and I am done serving fear. Help me to trust in You, and please make peace my portion.

Healing Testimony

Overcoming Multiple Allergies

I became chronically ill around the end of 2015 when I got mercury toxicity from eating way too much high-mercury fish. Once I was diagnosed and treated properly, I received some level of relief. From 2016 to 2020, I was treated at various medical and alternative clinics around the country, going up and down, always getting a new diagnosis, a new slew of supplements, medications, and treatments that were sure to lead to a complete healing, but never did. Over the years, I was diagnosed with Lyme disease, parasites, Epstein-Barr virus, mold toxicity, autoimmunity in the brain, MCS/EI, limbic system impairment, anxiety, mast cell activation syndrome, and more. For all those years, I hovered around 50 percent recovered. I was unable to work, but I could at least care for myself and participate in family functions and occasional fun activities.

In 2020, things took a bad turn. I kept getting worse with increasing sensitivities to sensory stimuli like computer screens, reading books, sounds from speakers, EMFs, even people's voices. It became increasingly severe to the point of being bedridden nearly all day. A year later, I finally surrendered and rededicated my life to Christ, and He immediately showed me some things to work on and within a few months, He led me to Be in Health. My parents were very helpful in trying to relay the teachings to me since I could not read, use a computer, or listen to sounds from speakers, and even talking was very limited. However, I was still resistant to what God was trying to show me.

Unbelievably, things got worse in 2022, and I was unable to tolerate even drinking water without a severe reaction. I ended up on hydration IVs to keep me alive for almost a year. A pastor prayed with me, and I was almost instantly healed of the sensitivity to people's voices, which allowed my parents to start reading God's Word to me. A friend and prayer partner referred the book *A More Excellent Way* by Dr. Henry W. Wright. I knew it was the Holy Spirit, and I finally relented.

My parents read Dr. Wright's book to me, and I began to understand the spiritual roots of all the various mental and physical maladies. We started to see some progress as we worked on the spiritual roots of multiple chemical sensitivity/environmental illness. As soon as we finished praying and repenting over my broken heart, not only was my heart healed but so was my body. I woke up the next day with the chills and body aches at least 50 percent reduced and significantly more energy. I learned firsthand the power and importance of repentance.

In August 2023, I went with my mom and dad to Thomaston, Georgia, for the For My Life Retreat and Walk Out Workshop. While I was there, I took back so many things! The sensitivity to sunlight was gone, I regained the ability to read and write with significantly less reaction, sensitivity to sounds from speakers was greatly reduced, and the sensitivity to smells was dramatically better.

Since returning home, I've been able to attend church, read God's Word, listen to praise and worship music, read other books, listen to teachings and podcasts on my phone and computer, talk on the phone, eat different foods, eat out at restaurants, drive my car, learn to play worship guitar, and many more things. Life is so much better! For the first time in my life, the thing I look forward to the most is growing closer to God.

One year ago, I was completely debilitated, lying in bed physically unable to do anything, not even drink water. And now I am a living testimony that miracles are still happening, and God is still healing people. I will be continuing on this journey of "walk out" until I am completely healed through the Father, the Son, and the Holy Spirit. Life is so good with Him!

—Nick

7

THE SPIRITUAL ROOTS OF AUTOIMMUNE DISEASE

Chapter Theme

We have discussed some of the steps necessary to restore our breakdown of relationship with Father God and with others, but what does it mean when we have separation from ourselves? The Old and New Testaments command us to love our neighbor as ourselves. What is the result when we not only struggle to love ourselves but have the enemy's evil thoughts tempting us to reject or even hate ourselves? The consequences of a breakdown in relationship with ourselves might be an autoimmune disease, which the medical community says is incurable and has an unknown etiology. The medical community does not have the answers, but we can trust that God and His Word can bring us freedom.

Questions for Reflection

1. Have you ever considered that you can have a breakdown in relationship with yourself?
2. Do you know people who struggle with self-hatred, self-rejection, and a belief that they are unlovable?
3. Have you considered that when you say you are unlovable, you are in rebellion and opposition against the Word of God?

Exploring Spiritual Roots

1. Is there a scriptural foundation for loving ourselves? (p. 121)

2. Often, individuals who are hard on themselves also have _____. This tendency leads them to _____. (p. 122)

3. The author has coined a term: the "unloving" spirit. What does it mean to be "unloving"? If someone is unable to receive love, _____. (p. 122)

4. An unloving spirit wants to protect the kingdom of self. Describe other traits of unloving spirits.

5. True love is not selfish. It does not _____. (p. 122) Love is self-less.

6. Self-rejection is a spiritual problem between each of us individually and Father God. With this problem, what do we refuse to believe? (pp. 122–123)

7. How do people searching for love judge themselves? (p. 123)

8. Where does our true value originate? We have value not because of our accomplishments but because _____. (p. 123)

9. What does a person with self-hatred believe? (p. 123)

10. How does self-hatred—an unloving spirit—negatively affect our immune system? If a person does not reject these thoughts from the enemy, the hypothalamus responds _____. The immune system weakens _____. (p. 123)

11. What is meant by an autoimmune disease? (p. 124)

12. The body attacks itself because the person is _____. As the person continues to attack himself or herself spiritually, the body finally agrees _____. (p. 124)

13. Quite literally, the body treats its own tissues as a foreign invader because _____. What has Satan persuaded them to believe? (pp. 123–124)

14. The author has concluded that most autoimmune diseases are the result of _____. (p. 124)

15. It could be said that autoimmune diseases are primarily a self-hatred disease _____. What are anxiety and stress a direct biological outcome of? (p. 124)

16. How can we accept ourselves? What does Psalm 139:14 say about our creation? (p. 124)

17. If we say that God does not love us or that we are unlovable, that is a work

_____ because we are in rebellion and opposition against the Word of

God. (p. 125)

18. What does self-rejection lead to? How does this make us a god unto ourselves? (pp. 125–126)

19. How does self-hatred often take hold in our life? Many cases of self-hatred begin with

_____. (p. 126)

20. How can we overcome self-hatred? (p. 127)

21. The truth is, we will make mistakes and fail in our journey as believers. What defines the difference
between the just man and the wicked man is not failure but

_____. Write out Proverbs 24:16.

(p. 127)

22. We all need to be loved. Instead of having our identity in the world, where must we find and accept
our identity? (p. 127)

23. What is the spiritual root cause of Type 1 diabetes? (p. 128)

24. The primary trigger point or spiritual root for lupus is _____ that defies a _____. (pp. 128–129)

25. The underlying spiritual root of rheumatoid arthritis is _____. The individual with RA doesn't accept themselves as they are and believes

_____. (p. 130)

26. Multiple sclerosis is deeply rooted in _____. As the person rejects their total identity, what questions do they ask? (p. 130)

27. Asking "Who cares?" is an orphan mentality. How can we overcome it? (p. 131)

28. What is the spiritual root cause of Crohn's disease? The individual is

_____. They become a false _____ and blame themselves for other's failures as well as their own. (p. 132)

29. What is the spiritual root cause of Graves' disease? This person takes on

_____. They may feel responsible for other people making the right _____ for their lives. (p. 133)

30. The author believes the antidote to self-hatred and autoimmune disorders is embracing the truth of

_____. (p. 136)

Applying Principles of Healing

Conclusion

Autoimmune diseases have mystified the field of medicine since their earliest diagnoses. Without any strong evidence of the root causes, physicians turn to adjusting the patient's environment or prescribing new drugs to manage the disease. However, God has a better answer through exposing the spiritual roots of autoimmune diseases. A disease of self-hate or self-rejection results when you do not accept who you are in creation. Guilt and shame follow you. You're always looking over your shoulder for somebody else's approval and not getting it. But you have a Father, and you can embrace the principles of life. Be in Health has seen countless people healed of autoimmune disorders after repenting of self-hatred, self-rejection, and guilt, and coming into agreement with God's Word that they are loved and accepted apart from performance and expectations of others.

Thinking It Over

1. You are not rejected by God, so why are you rejecting yourself?
2. What happens when you argue with the Word of God that declares He has accepted you?
3. Are you ready to take ownership of your life and to have life more abundantly?

Acting on It

1. If you have an autoimmune disease, read Psalm 139 daily. Meditate on the many verses that speak of God's love for you. Embrace the truth of the thoughts God has toward you in this psalm.
2. Repent of hating and rejecting yourself to this God who loves you.
3. Stop self-accusation and arguing with God.
4. Remind yourself, "I may have a disease, but I am not a disease!" Don't call it "my disease." There is sin that has been tormenting you, but you are not the sin. You are a child of God! Accept the Father's great love for you; He has called you to be His own!

Praying Over It

Father God, thank You for loving me and not rejecting me. I'm sorry for rejecting myself. And thank You for forgiving me. I embrace Jesus's work for me on the cross and receive forgiveness. His death was sufficient to free me from who I am and what I have done wrong. I don't want to have anything between You and me. Help me to have my identity fully in You and Your Word and not based upon anything I do or anyone else's expectations of me. Help me to love myself the way You love me. And thank You for Your declarations that I am fearfully and wonderfully made. I agree with Your Word!

Healing Testimony

My Victory Over Autoimmune Disease

In June 2023, I had my annual physical, and my liver enzymes were way above normal. I was sent to a specialist who ordered a liver biopsy. The results were an autoimmune liver disease. When I heard those words, I knew the Lord could heal me. The doctor prescribed high doses of prednisone and another drug with so many risk factors that I declined to take it. Instead, I asked the doctor to let me do the prednisone treatment and then see how my enzyme numbers were after stopping the prednisone. I knew the prednisone would give me the time to look deeply into my heart for what I needed to do with the Lord.

God took me on a journey that started by watching *Real Solutions for Autoimmune Disease* by Pastors John and Adrienne Shales. This teaching helped me understand the deep root causes of autoimmune disease, and it brought back Father God's love for me that I had forgotten. My time was filled with prayer and conversations with God, getting down deep into the roots that were causing my infirmity. The fear, shame, guilt, self-hatred, self-bitterness, and unloving spirits had to be removed from my heart and life. The Shales said something that has stuck with me: "I had been trained by the enemy from birth to be a slave to his every lie. My heavenly Father had plans to give me His perfect love and abundant life." I had to trust Him, which began a new life for me living in God's kingdom on earth. I was learning to trust, trust, trust my heavenly Father in the midst of the enemy's relentless lies. He doesn't give up easily—he had lied to me for seventy-three years. I learned it is so important to know who is speaking to me and to shut off the enemy's voice with God's Word, just like Jesus did when Satan came to tempt Him.

I started this journey in June, trusting I would be healed as I dealt with the possible spiritual roots that brought autoimmune disease. I had several fruitful Spiritual Lifeline appointments, pulled the diagnosis down in Jesus's name, and allowed the Holy Spirit to guide me through the 8 Rs for every spiritual stronghold I needed to get out of my life. I received the Father's love to overflowing, and I forgave myself. This was not a "process" but a renewed *relationship* with my heavenly Father that I had missed for thirty years. The Father, Jesus, and the Holy Spirit have always been a part of my life, but they were not given their supernatural throne in my world. Through the teachings at Be in Health, the truth of God's kingdom was brought back into my heart.

I finished with prednisone treatments in mid-August and took another blood test at the end of September, enough time for the prednisone to be out of my system. On October 2, the doctor gave me the good news that my numbers were all normal. I cried with joy and praised the Lord for His healing. When I saw the doctor, I gave him *Exposing the Spiritual Roots of Disease* by Dr. Henry W. Wright. I told him that God healed me, and he said he would read the book.

—Kris

8

THE SPIRITUAL ROOTS OF CARDIOVASCULAR DISEASE

Chapter Theme

Heart disease is still the number one killer in America. According to the American Heart Association, in recent years, cardiovascular disease has accounted for nearly 840,000 deaths each year in the U.S. Why is this happening? The Bible speaks often about the significance of the heart. Proverbs 4:23 says, *"Keep thy heart with all diligence; for out of it are the issues of life."* What flows from our heart? Physically, our heart is the organ that pumps the blood of life through our bodies. Spiritually, the heart is the central residence of our spirit. We need to learn to guard our heart and protect the very issue (source) of our life. We have the blessing of health when we are walking in obedience to God's Word.

Questions for Reflection

1. Do you see any cardiovascular issues or health problems in your family history that you might recognize as a generational vulnerability through a genetic component?

2. If you have a sickness or disease, is that evidence that these principles do not work or is it evidence that you are an imperfect human and not sinless?

3. What does it mean to say we are a "work in progress?"

Exploring Spiritual Roots

1. The conventional methods for preventing cardiovascular disease primarily focus on

   _____. Moderation, or _____, is good to practice

   when it comes to certain foods because your body is _____. (p. 141)

2. Why does Scripture say that exercise "profits little"? Nutrition and exercise won't replace

_____. (p. 141)

3. What did the author need to do after his heart attack? (p. 143)

4. Write out some of these Scriptures that the author held so that he would not become hopeless: Nehemiah 8:10; Proverbs 17:22; Psalm 118:17.

5. Some people resign themselves to death and believe _____. But to equate aging with death is to _____. In the kingdom of God, there is no such thing as retirement. You serve others, and _____! (p. 148)

6. List the major, underlying spiritual roots of heart disease. (p. 148)

7. The author has observed that people who embrace anger and rage as a lifestyle are susceptible to heart disease. What are some demonstrations of that type of anger? (p. 151)

8. Anger and rage begin with _____

_____. Among other things, they lead to _____. Ongoing hostility brings with it an avalanche of stress hormones that

_____. (p. 151)

9. Be in Health has found that Type A personalities have a greater tendency toward anger.

   Cardiologists recognize that Type A personalities are _____. Are these traits listed as fruit of the Holy Spirit? (p. 151)

10. By contrast, what is a list of the fruits of the Holy Spirit according to Galatians 5:22–23? (p. 151)

11. How can someone break away from the addiction to strong emotions like fear, anger, and rage? Your addiction is _____. (p. 152)

12. In many families, lashing out in anger and rage is a _____. Some people may feel vulnerable and afraid if _____. But faith toward God _____. (p. 152)

13. We must know the truth of God's Word in order to be free. To keep from becoming frustrated in situations or from lashing out in anger and rage toward others, what must we embrace? What do we need to repent of? (pp. 152–153)

14. Because of the spirit-soul-body connection, the Lord is concerned with both the spiritual and the physical hardening of our hearts. What warning do we read in Psalm 95:8? (p. 153)

15. What does it mean to harden your heart? What warning does Hebrews 3:12 give us? (p. 153)

16. A hard heart is also the result of a spirit of _____, which is not

    _____. (p. 153)

17. Allow the love and peace of God _____.

    _____ to a hardened heart. (p. 153)

18. With heart problems, people have _____. Jesus offers us His peace that is beyond any other the world can offer. To have that kind of peace, what should we do? Write Jesus's promise from John 14:27. (p. 154)

19. Luke 21:16 says that in the last days, men's hearts _____. What are many people afraid of today? What is the opposite of fear and stress? (pp. 154–155)

20. The author has observed that the first target organ for the spiritual roots of fear is _____. Remember, the enemy cannot give us a cardiovascular disease just by tempting us with thoughts unless _____. (p. 155)

21. When we are tempted by fear, we must make a decision to _____. We can take on _____ and repent of _____. (p. 155)

22. What are the spiritual roots of high blood pressure? What does the Word tells us in Matthew 6:34? (p. 156)

23. Angina pectoris stems from _____, as God's Word says, *"Men's hearts failing them for fear* (Luke 21:26). The spirit of fear also makes them feel like _____. (p. 157)

24. What is the spiritual root of heart arrhythmias? This person strives to be _____. (p. 157)

25. Mitro valve prolapse condition stems from _____ with the manifestation of _____. These individuals feel as though _____. (p. 158)

26. What is the spiritual root of aneurysms, and what do they reveal? They dwell on thoughts of _____. (pp. 158–159)

27. What does coronary artery disease stem from? It is a love issue from _____. (p. 159)

28. The spiritual root of cardiomyopathy is having _____ that is consumed with _____. These individuals may struggle with _____. (p. 160)

29. As you have seen, it is vital for our heart health that we cease from anger. Psalm 103:8 tells us,

_____. This is your road map to learning to partake of God's nature and to be free from heart disease. (p. 160)

Applying Principles of Healing

Conclusion

When you bring God into the equation of heart health, everything changes for the better. If you are suffering from heart disease or are a likely candidate for it in the future, Father God wants to change your course direction. You need to make daily decisions to follow the Word of God in obedience. Even when you are tempted to focus on and become fearful or enraged by a bad circumstance, you must make the decision to choose Father God instead. We live in this world, but we don't have to act like the world. Take on God's nature instead. Repent of, and put off, Satan's nature, which is creating disease in your body. Win this physical and spiritual battle in your life!

Thinking It Over

1. The Word warns us, *"Be not hasty in thy spirit to be angry: for anger resteth in the bosom of fools"* (Ecclesiastes 7:9). Have there been times in your life where you have been stirred up by anger and only looked foolish?

2. The Bible also says, *"He that hath no rule over his own spirit is like a city that is broken down, and without walls"* (Proverbs 25:28). When you feel angry and have thoughts of the offenses done to you, do you take time to pause and consider where these thoughts of offenses are coming from? Do you rule your own spirit or are the walls of your city broken down?

3. Are you ready to take responsibility for your life, deal with your iniquity, and become an overcomer?

Acting on It

1. If your earthly father treated you poorly or neglected you, do not continue to hold a grudge toward him. It is time to repent to Father God for bitterness and anger toward your father and forgive him. This is how we end the cycle.

2. Forgive others in spite of the offense against you. Proverbs 19:11 says, *"The discretion of a man deferreth his anger; and it is his glory to pass over a transgression."* Read this verse often. The more you practice releasing to Father God any transgressions done against you, the less power Satan's kingdom has to tempt you.

3. Purpose to keep a soft and open heart to the Lord and His voice.

4. Make daily decisions to follow the Word of God in obedience, instead of becoming fearful of a bad circumstance. You must make these decisions moment by moment and day by day.

Pray About It

Father, thank You for Your Word, which takes us beyond science to the full truth. Thank You for warning us that anger, rage, hostility, stress, fear, anxiety, and hard-heartedness can have a direct impact on our cardiovascular health. God, You are greater than our sin. First John 3:20 says, *"For if our heart condemn us, God is greater than our heart, and knoweth all things."* Therefore, Lord, even if our heart condemns us, You are greater than our sin. And if we confess our sins and repent of them, Your Holy Spirit will help us with a reformation in our personalities. In Jesus's name, amen.

Healing Testimony

Victory Over High Blood Pressure

Over the course of a few years, whenever I'd go in for a checkup, the doctor would tell me that my blood pressure was slightly elevated. At the time, I didn't think much about it because it had always been the perfect 120/80, so slightly elevated wasn't too big a deal.

I had noticed that I was having severe headaches weekly to the point that I was becoming sick, and it would take around two days for the headache to fully go away. I stopped taking acetaminophen or ibuprofen when I would get them because nothing would help except time. I figured it was better to not take anything than to continuously take something that wasn't going to help either way. My mother would ask me whether I had checked my blood pressure because high blood pressure ran in our family and it could be why I was having such severe headaches. I did check it and realized that it was extremely high. I continued to monitor it over the course of the next few weeks. It remained high, but I was trying to manage the symptoms without actually addressing the real issue.

On a Sunday afternoon in the summer of 2020, I was extremely sick and discovered that my blood pressure was 186/116, so I went to the emergency room. At first, the doctor wanted to rule out anything neurological; since I was in my early thirties, he felt it was unlikely that I had high blood pressure. After many tests, he did determine that my blood pressure was indeed high.

My life had become very hectic, and I was taking on a lot that wasn't mine to take on, but I felt like it was my job. I started talking to God and telling Him that I did not want to be on this medication for the rest of my life, even though the enemy really tried to tell me that that was what my life was now, to be managed by this medication so that I could be *normal*. I really wanted to be free from this. Thankfully, I knew of a place that could help me realize what was going on in my life.

I have been through For My Life many times, I worked at Be in Health for almost ten years and knew the information for many different possible spiritual roots; however, I was not fully walking in what I knew as truth. I had always heard the possible spiritual roots for high blood pressure to be fear of tomorrow or dread, which were prevalent in my life, but I didn't fully take that in as the cause. I knew there was something more because as much as I prayed for revelation for the fear and dread, nothing seemed to have the breakthrough for me to be healed from the high blood pressure.

During the summer of 2024, I had a long talk with God and told Him that I wanted to be free and healed from this because I did not want to continue living this way. I felt in my spirit that He was telling me that if I would just truly listen, He would give me the answer and I would walk away healed. I went to the For My Life Retreat that June, and the day I received the diagnosis sheet with the possible spiritual roots, I saw something that I had never seen before. Now, it was probably always there, but the enemy really blinded me to it because he wanted to keep me in bondage. What I saw was the spiritual root of *anger*! That was it. I knew then that was what had been keeping me in bondage. Generational rage and anger was strong in my family line, and it had been a part of who I was growing up and into adulthood. The thing God showed me that week was that I was getting angry over things that I could not control, things that were not my responsibility but that I had taken on and taken in as mine when they really weren't. Then when the outcome wasn't what I thought it should be, I would become angry—angry at others and angry at myself.

I began to understand that in the areas where I was getting upset, I wasn't truly trusting God. If I had complete faith and trust in God, knowing that all things work together for good according to His purpose, it doesn't matter what the outcome is, *He* has it under control. That's it, end of discussion.

What God uncovered was that in the areas where I was getting upset, I was feeling like a failure, and I would get upset at myself because I thought that I could do better, even though I had done all that I could. I believed that my identity and worth were in what I was doing and if I failed, that I was a failure and was worth nothing to anyone. I would then get angry at myself and go into drivenness and performance to make sure that it would get done perfectly. This would also lead me to lash out at others when things were not done the way I thought they should be done or in the timeframe I thought they should be completed.

After that week, I was able to come off all my medications. The first week after I was off them, the enemy tried to come in and tempt me by telling me that I was not healed and that I would be on the medication for the rest of my life. This was the biggest lie ever! I've been off the medication fully since July and have not had any issues with my blood pressure at all. Do I still get upset and angry? Yes. Do I allow the enemy to make me stew over my problems like I did before? No! That is the difference. If I get upset, that is okay. I'm only human. I am not perfect, and I'll make mistakes, but I don't have to focus on them.

—Mary

9

THE SPIRITUAL ROOTS OF MENTAL ILLNESS

Chapter Theme

Diseases of the mind begin the same way as other diseases. The enemy begins to infiltrate your thoughts with temptations and lies from within. When you embrace those lies as truth instead of believing the Word of God, your mind will be affected. If you have been born again, you should have joy because of your relationship with the Godhead. After all, as believers, we all have the joy of the Lord as our strength! (See Nehemiah 8:10.) Then why do some Christians struggle with hopelessness, depression, and despair? Throughout this study, you have learned that you are a triune being— you are a spirit, you have a soul, and you live in a body. This is a foundational truth for the healing of all disease, including mental illness. Your spirituality directly affects every part of your physical body, and that includes your brain. It's time to uncover the spiritual roots of disease that can affect the mind.

Questions for Reflection

1. Have you, or a loved one, ever struggled with hopelessness or a sadness that you couldn't seem to overcome?

2. Do you understand that all the enemy needs to do is to manipulate your biochemistry through thought? In the case of depression, your brain has conformed to those thoughts.

3. Have you considered that the Word of God has the power to lift you from the darkness of depression?

Exploring Spiritual Roots

1. Depression is defined as a mental health disorder that involves a person's thoughts, behavior, feelings, and sense of well-being. Describe some of the feelings of a depressed man or woman. (p. 166)

2. Biologically, depression is defined as _____. There is nothing wrong with the brain, but there is a disruption _____. What is the result of a disruption of homeostasis in the brain over time? (p. 166)

3. Science says that depression comes from a combination of factors. What are those factors? (pp. 166–167)

4. What is one area that science never acknowledges as a factor in diseases of the mind? (p. 167)

5. When addressing depression, scientists focus on counseling _____. In contrast, Be in Health focuses on _____. (p. 167)

6. List three specific spiritual roots behind depression. (p. 167)

7. What does the spirit of self-accusation accuse the person of? What do the spirits of self-introspection and self-centeredness cause the person to focus on? (p. 167)

8. _____ makes a person feel devalued. _____ will not allow them to believe that they can be forgiven for their sin. _____ is the glue that binds all these spirits together. The author calls self-pity _____ binding a person to their past (failures). Self-pity relives the failure in the past by _____. (p. 167)

9. Serotonin is also depleted in individuals who _____. This affects the hypothalamus and other glands that are responsible for _____ _____. (p. 168)

10. Practitioners recommend forms of mindless meditation to gain peace over anxiety and stress. This is _____ teaching. What does mindless meditation open the door to? (p. 168)

11. What is biblical meditation? Write Psalm 119:15. (p. 168)

12. Serotonin reuptake inhibitors (SSRIs) redirect a person's consciousness so that they are now unaware of _____. But even if we block the pathways to depression, _____. (p. 169)

13. What does God want us to do instead of going into an altered state of consciousness? (p. 169)

14. What does the author mean by the phrase "take ownership of your life?" (p. 170)

15. Remember this truth, *"So then faith cometh by hearing, and hearing by the word of God"* (Romans 10:17). There is a battle over each of us every day. What is our role in the battle? What should we saturate our mind with daily? (p. 170)

16. Name several things that will bring our serotonin level back into balance. (pp. 170–171)

17. A person's mind may have been trained in hopelessness and despair for some time. They will need to _____. (p. 172)

18. An important first step to recovery is _____. Depression will isolate us from people when we need them the most because _____. (p. 172)

19. Name another powerful tool for defeating depression. The power of the _____ and our _____ can defeat depression in our lives. (p. 173)

20. In addition to heredity, the spiritual root of bipolar disorder comes from generations of an unloving spirit, where the individuals do not _____ _____. The physical response to this unloving spirit is a reduction of serotonin. (pp. 173–174)

21. How can someone recover from bipolar disorder? As they hear and dwell on God's Word, His voice _____ and the voice of the enemy _____. The neurotransmitter imbalances will return to normal. (p. 174)

22. _____ is the spiritual root behind paranoid schizophrenia. Those who develop this condition generally grew up in families that _____. The fight-or-flight response can begin in a young person who does not feel safe in their family because of _____. (p. 174)

23. To help people who are struggling with their identity and have depressive episodes, including paranoid schizophrenia, we should _____. Write 1 John 4:18: (p. 175)

24. What has the author found that post-traumatic stress disorder (PTSD) involves? What happens if someone who already has an enlarged amygdala arrives in a war zone? (p. 177)

25. What do sufferers of PTSD need to do to become free? (p. 177)

26. What are the spiritual roots behind obsessive-compulsive disorder (OCD)? This individual believes they cannot be forgiven _____. In addition, they have _____ that beats them up for these same failures. (p. 179)

27. What is the path of freedom for a person with OCD? (p. 179)

28. Many people are filled with _____ and it has often been years since they have _____. Even salvation has not been a joy to them because they have lived _____. (p. 179)

Applying Principles of Healing

Conclusion

Having the mind of Christ is the key to mental health. Our lives depend on being willing and able to be changed. God will continue to change us, but we must understand our responsibility. There is power in God's Word. Don't be afraid of this battle. God's thinking is superior, and Satan's thinking is inferior. *"Ye are of God, little children, and have overcome them: because greater is he that is in you, than he that is in the world"* (1 John 4:4). Greater is God who is in you than the enemy who is in the world. You must choose whom you will serve. God will not leave you nor forsake you as you take this journey to freedom!

Thinking It Over

1. After doing this study, what would you say to someone whom you suspect is suffering from depression?
2. Were you surprised to hear the results of the 3-year scientific PHYMSH study of the people who attended the For My Life Retreat?
3. Has the enemy had you under a burden of accusation? Repent of believing him and renew the joy of your salvation!

Acting on It

1. If you have struggled with mental illness, read Hebrews 4:12. Believe that the Word of God has the power to divide between your soul and your spirit and bring God's truth into your depressed state.
2. Repent of accepting thoughts and feelings that are not based on God's Word. Consider God's Word daily instead.
3. Pray and meditate on Nehemiah 8:10. *"Then he said unto them, Go your way, eat the fat, and drink the sweet, and send portions unto them for whom nothing is prepared: for this day is holy unto our Lord: neither be ye sorry; for the joy of the Lord is your strength."*
4. Step out of isolation and surround yourself with those who love you.

Praying About It

According to Psalm 51:12, Lord, restore unto me the joy of Your salvation. Thank You for the truth of this joy that comes from You. Thank You that the kingdom of God is not meat and drink, but righteousness, peace, and joy in the Holy Spirit. (See Romans 14:17.) Joy in the Holy Spirit is for me! Thank You that greater are You within me than the enemy that is in the world. (See 1 John 4:4.) Thank You that You never leave me nor forsake me. (See Hebrews 13:5.)

Healing Testimony

Defeating Depression

I never thought I'd be writing a testimony of defeating depression. I was told and believed that I would be dealing with it all my life. The prognosis was clear: I would have good days and bad days; I would have to work hard every day to get out of bed; and I would always have to take medication. This would be my normal. I was just a depressed person—that was my identity.

I was diagnosed with major depression, along with anorexia nervosa and generalized anxiety disorder, around the age of fourteen years old. Almost immediately, I was put on a very strong SSRI (selective serotonin reuptake inhibitor) medication. I experienced negative side effects that led to doctors prescribing a less serious medication at a high dosage instead. I continued therapy regularly over the next few years.

Eventually, I started using recreational drugs along with the medication to fight off the depression that still ran rampant. When I started a spiritual journey into New Age and paganism, drug use was encouraged to expand my mind and spirit. The drug use, compounded with the chemical imbalance created by my medications, led to a severe adverse reaction, sending me into a deep depressive psychosis. This happened twice within a year, and each time, doctors were uncertain about my recovery. But I had a very significant experience of Christ.

It wasn't until I heard about the principles taught in the For My Life Retreat that I considered what I had heard about the Bible and Christianity might not be the strict and hateful religion that some made it out to be. At every turn, For My Life explained with Scripture why medication, drugs, Reiki, or "enlightenment" never worked. I was so amazed that all of this was in the Bible. It flipped the script for how I viewed God, Jesus, the Bible—everything. I realized that I needed to be free of the self-pity and rejection I had continued to live in that kept that depression around.

A few weeks after the retreat, I ran out of my medication and was due to see my psychiatrist for a refill. Usually, after missing a daily dose, I would have horrible side effects, but I noticed that the side effects were nonexistent. It was divine timing, as I told my doctor. He said that since I had been doing better, I could try living without the medication and see how things went. I've never had to call him back!

By allowing the Spirit of God into my life and filling up with the Word, depression is gone from my life. I realize now that a large part of my struggle was a lack of identity—not knowing who I really was or could be instead of being a depressed person. God had so much more for me, and He still does!

—Jenn

10

THE SPIRITUAL ROOTS OF STRESS DISORDERS

Chapter Theme

There is an excessive amount of stress in America, affecting over forty million adults. Anxiety disorders are the most common mental illness in the U.S., and three-fourths of employees believe that workers today have more on-the-job stress than a generation ago. And in many cultures, there is a demand for perfection. This creates a lot of stress and anxiety in people's lives. When they internalize this stress, it starts to affect their soul and many of their bodily systems. Stress disorders, or syndromes, are a result of a spirit of fear (which manifests as anxiety and stress), along with guilt and shame. With stress disorders, the enemy produces fearful thoughts that cause you to lose your peace. As you dwell on those thoughts, your central nervous system is affected. Medication will only mask these chemical imbalances, which come as a result of embracing a spirit of fear. Remember that today's society may not make provision for failure, but God always does!

Questions for Reflection

1. Are you trying to receive healing despite rebellion against the Word of God?
2. Were you surprised to hear that 80 to 90 percent of people have indicated to the author that they never heard their father say, "I love you?"
3. Can you say that you are anxious for nothing as it says in Philippians 4:6?

Exploring Spiritual Roots

1. How does Satan tempt us in our thoughts to convince us to speak against ourselves?

   _____. What is an example of that kind of thought? (pp. 184–185)

2. Why does unresolved fear make it impossible to have a sound mind? Individuals with fear have trouble _____ love in relationships. (p. 185)

3. If someone didn't feel loved during their childhood, they probably _____. What joins itself to a person who was not loved correctly? (p. 185)

4. Write Proverbs 29:25. What is the "fear of man?" We must declare Hebrews 13:6, which says: _____. (p. 185)

5. If someone has a fear of others, they need to trust Father God to _____. Where is the one place we can go to learn how to trust and love other people again? It is the one place we should be _____. (p. 186)

6. What is the author's definition of a disease? (p. 186)

7. In contrast, what is the author's definition of a syndrome? Stress disorders are _____. (p. 186)

8. Medical science has observed that _____, but they do not know the cure. What does the author state is the cure? Then God's truth will become a part of your _____, replacing the stress-filled lies of the enemy with peace that will reign in your heart. (p. 187)

9. Fibromyalgia often affects women who _____. It primarily comes from

_____ by a man. A spirit of

_____ comes into their lives. This spirit of fear produces

_____. (p. 190)

10. To be healed of fibromyalgia, the individual must repent of embracing the spirit of fear

of abandonment _____. They may need to repent of

_____, as well. When peace returns, the nerve signal calms down.
(p. 191)

11. The spiritual root of chronic fatigue syndrome (CFS) is a _____ and

behind it is a _____, usually a parent. (p. 192)

12. The cure for CFS is to repent, release that drive _____, and realize

_____. This person does not have to _____. God always accepts

them. We should not look to ourselves or others _____. God is our source.
(p. 192)

13. What is the spiritual root of Type 2 diabetes? They look to others _____.

It is also linked to obesity, so eating _____. (p. 193)

14. We must all learn that our acceptance and _____. He is enough.
We must embrace the foundational Scripture for the healing of stress disorders, 1 John 4:18:

_____ (p. 194)

15. All spiritually rooted disease caused by fear _____ with God, ourselves, or others. How do we know there is still unforgiveness, bitterness, or hatred in our heart toward another? (p. 194)

16. Irritable bowel syndrome (IBS) is produced by _____ primarily in women who were _____. (p. 195)

17. _____, not the mother, is responsible for the emotional well-being of his daughter. Many homes have been destroyed through _____. If a man does not believe he is loved by Father God, _____. (p. 195)

18. What may happen after we have negative experiences with our earthly father? To overcome this serious spiritual defect, what must we do? (p. 196)

19. What is the spiritual root of both ulcerative colitis (UC) and malabsorption, or leaky gut syndrome? What is the cure for UC? (p. 196)

20. Acid reflux, or heartburn, and gastroesophageal reflux disease (GERD) are brought on by _____. This person is unsure _____. Its armor includes: _____. The person must repent of harboring _____ and spirits of fear. (p. 197)

21. Migraines have two spiritual roots: _____ about _____. The external conflict _____. The internal conflict _____. (p. 198)

22. The author's prescription for migraines is _____ that is tormenting them, and that they take _____ and _____. (p. 198)

23. What is the spiritual root of chronic insomnia? We need to _____ despite not knowing the outcome and _____. (p. 198)

24. Simple acne has a spiritual root _____. Repent of these fears and make a decision _____. (pp. 198–199)

25. Asthma is a stress disorder that is the product of a specific root issue: _____. The antidote is God's promise that _____. (p. 199)

26. What are the spiritual roots behind an overeating disorder? It is also an _____, rooted in a need to be loved. Instead of choosing food as comfort, this person needs to _____. (p. 199)

27. What must we do to be truly healed and free? (p. 200)

28. We need to guard against _____ and remember that we are

_____. How we handle the temptation will

_____. (p. 200)

Applying Principles of Healing

Conclusion

If you are struggling with a stress disorder, you are not alone in the battle! The Holy Spirit will help you to "walk out" of Satan's kingdom one day at a time in the areas where you have allowed sin to rule your decision-making. As you repent of sin, you are choosing to serve Him and walking into the blessings of Father God's kingdom instead. God loves you, and He has good things planned for your life—not rejection, fear, or stress disorders. Let Him transform your mind with His Word because your spirituality impacts your health in every dimension!

Thinking It Over

1. What fears in your life might you need to face and defeat?

2. Is your value established alone by God? Do you believe you are fearfully and wonderfully made according to Psalm 139:14?

3. Do you *believe* that Father God is saying you are His beloved son or daughter in whom He is well pleased?

Acting on It

1. Learn to trust in God and His love to repair and bring healing to those parts of your life where you have felt alone and abandoned. *"Cast all your care upon him; for he careth for you"* (1 Peter 5:7).

2. Renew your mind with biblical truth so you never again embrace the law of sin concerning fear of abandonment and anxiety. As it says in Isaiah 26:3, *"Thou will keep him in perfect pace, whose mind is stayed on thee: because he trusteth in thee."*

3. If your healing does not occur instantly after you repent to Father God, set your face like flint and determine to follow the Word of God regardless of what you feel. Draw a line in the sand and say, "No further with the lies, Satan, in Jesus's name!"

Praying About It

Father, thank You that I am Your child, and You are well pleased with me. I am so grateful that You alone establish my value and identity so that I never have to earn it or be afraid of what others think of me or what they may do to me. Thank You that I don't have to carry all the burdens I have been carrying. Thank You that I can trust You even if I don't know the outcome. Thank You that You never leave me nor forsake me. Thank You for being a loving and good Father and for bringing peace to every part of my body. I rest in You.

Healing Testimony

Victory Over Stress Disorders

Prior to attending a For My Life Retreat, my life was marred by a series of health challenges. I struggled with a weakened immune system, an array of allergies, psoriasis, hemorrhoids, and extensive gastrointestinal issues, including complications with my kidneys, gallbladder, intestines, liver, and spleen. I also had diagnoses of severe depression, anxiety, PTSD, and PMDD, as well as experiencing suicidal ideations and symptoms associated with schizophrenia. I struggled with doing normal daily things like going to the bathroom, working, and even going to church. At night, it was the worst. I suffered with intense night terrors, tormenting nightmares, insomnia, and sleep paralysis. I lived in a victim mindset. How can a Christian deal with such trauma and pain?

In 2023, my aunt gave me the book *Exposing the Spiritual Roots of Disease* by Dr. Henry W. Wright. I couldn't believe what I was reading! In December of that year, the Lord opened a door for me and my aunt to attend the week-long retreat at Be in Health called the City of Refuge. Two days into the conference, I was experiencing serious pain in my side and when going to the bathroom. However, on the third day, I recognized the sin in my life and began taking responsibility for what God was revealing to me. As I repented and renounced the sin, God showed His victory in my life, and I was healed!

Since applying the Be in Health teachings, I have had life-changing results! I have a better understanding of the root causes of disease. I understand the Word more clearly. My relationship with God has grown tremendously, and my relationships with family and friends have grown as well. These biblical truths have completely changed how I view life. They have helped me to reach out to believers and unbelievers alike. I'm now able to discern whether my thoughts are of God or of the enemy. The For My Life Retreat deepened my relationship with my heavenly Father, increased my faith, delivered me from the enemy, and gave me tools to overcome in the very real spiritual war. I was healed of every condition I had after I arrived at Be in Health. The peace I now experience is indescribable, and I feel incredibly blessed!

—Deenah

11

WHAT'S NEXT?

Chapter Theme

As you have seen throughout this study, spiritually rooted disease is a result of separation from God, separation from yourself, or separation from others. All healing of spiritually rooted disease begins with reconciliation with God—receiving His love, embracing Him as your Father, and making your peace with Him. There are two kingdoms waging war on the inside of you: the law of sin and the law of God. God will not live your life for you! Once you are delivered from evil roots, it becomes your responsibility to renew your mind and change those old patterns of ungodly thinking, casting down evil imaginations, and filling yourself with the Word of God in your thought life. While the world might be struggling in disease and hopelessness, you should be a happy, well-balanced, and enthusiastic son or daughter of God. God wants you to walk in and rejoice in your freedom!

Questions for Reflection

1. How has this study changed your perception of the true cause and cure of disease? Have you learned that you are not your disease?

2. Has this study helped you uncover any negative thoughts that Satan repeats to you that are against God's Word? If so, have you recognized the answer to his attacks against you?

3. How might you apply this knowledge to your life in the future?

Exploring Spiritual Roots

1. How do we renew our minds and change those old patterns of ungodly thinking? (pp. 205–206)

2. Why does Be in Health call this process to freedom "Walk Out?" (p. 206)

3. What do we need to do in addition to being prayed for? (p. 206)

4. What does John 8:32 declare? (p. 206)

5. What type of people does the following Scripture refer to: *"Ever learning, and never able to come to the knowledge of the truth"* (2 Timothy 3:7)? How must we be led instead? (p. 206)

6. How do we have the power to be free from disease? Our freedom was paid for _____ and the power of God so that we could live in freedom. (p. 206)

7. How does God train us in righteousness? Write Psalm 1:2.

8. How do we dwell on God's Word? We take a Scripture verse or passage and not merely read it once _____. We take in the Word, _____ _____. In that way, God's Word becomes a part of _____. (pp. 206–207)

9. What is Satan's counterfeit to dwelling on God's Word? (p. 207)

10. Father God desires for us to be free from conforming to the world by doing what? Write out Romans 12:1–2. (pp. 207–208)

11. Our mind becomes renewed by being _____ with the washing of the water of the Word: *"That he might sanctify and cleanse it* [the church] *with the washing of water by the word"* (Ephesians 5:26). (p. 208)

12. When we meditate on God's Word day and night, we _____. A renewed mind is now able to _____. (p. 208)

13. Renewing our minds in God's Word _____. This is how we become spiritual people in how _____. (p. 208)

14. The journey of _____ helps us know how God wants us to think and apply it to our lives. (p. 208)

15. We need to face our fears, our anxieties, and our sins. We are supposed to be changed from _____ because that is Satan's domain. As a result, you will be _____. (p. 208)

16. What happens if someone thinks the work is too hard and wants to just take a pill? (p. 208)

17. What is the daily requirement in Philippians 2:12? (p. 208)

18. What are two temptations that people might embrace after they hear the truth of these teachings? (p. 209)

19. We were not called to be one of God's own _____; we were called _____! (p. 209)

20. People with unbelief will try to _____ to their image. We are not being formed _____. We are being transformed _____! (p. 209)

21. Write out the truth of 2 Corinthians 3:18. (p. 209)

22. What can we expect as we are being changed into the Lord's image? (p.209)

23. Through Jesus Christ, the Father is _____ in the tragedy of the garden of Eden, _____.That is the _____. (p. 209)

24. According to 1 Peter 2:19, we are being called out of darkness and _____. (p. 209)

25. It may feel uncomfortable to confront certain issues brought up in this teaching, but the author implores you to address them because _____ _____. (p. 210)

Applying Principles of Healing

Conclusion

Do not let anyone tell you that you're not the apple of God's eye. (See Deuteronomy 32:10.) Do not let anybody tell you that you are not engraved in the palm of His hands. (See Isaiah 49:16.) Do not let anyone tell you that your name is not written down in the Book of Life (see, for example, Revelation 3:5), or that you are not a son or daughter of the Father (see, for example, Galatians 4:6). Don't let anyone interfere with who you are. You are not an accident; you were a planned event by God. Before you were ever conceived, God knew you; before your body parts began to form, He said, *"You are mine"* (Isaiah 43:1). God has created you with a purpose and a plan, and He has created you to live!

Thinking It Over

1. Are you ready to take this journey of being changed from the inside out so that your diseases vanish? God promises to be there with you!

2. As you've read God's Word in this study, will you truly embrace the truth of how much Father God loves you?

3. Do you believe that God has given you the power of the Holy Spirit to help you in the task of changing your thought patterns forever?

Acting on It

1. Relax in the Father's love. Breathe in and breathe out. Let God renew you.

2. Stop listening to the devil.

3. Be kind to yourself.

4. Choose life and not death.

Praying About It

Father, I have listened to lies that I didn't know were lies. I have pursued things I thought were right but lead to my destruction. Please continue to show me the good way where there is rest for my soul. Mature me as Your child. Let me be whole in spirit, soul, and body, and may the generations after me also be whole so that the world may see Your glory, goodness, and love toward us. Continue to teach me by Your grace. Thank You, Father, for Your love, for the sacrifice of Jesus Christ Your Son on my behalf, and for the power of the Holy Spirit that leads and guides me through my journey to health and wholeness.

WHAT BE IN HEALTH® OFFERS

Now that you've read this study guide, you may be interested in these other resources that Be in Health has to offer.

The Overcomers' Community® Partners

The journey of being an overcomer can be challenging, and we don't want you to have to do it alone. That is why we've developed the Overcomers' Community Partners. The OC Partnership is an opportunity for you to participate with and be plugged into Be in Health on an ongoing basis. It is the only place available for you to receive ongoing, interactive discipleship from Be in Health team members and a large community of other believers around the world who are in the walk-out journey alongside you. You may participate in weekly online groups, have access to our spiritual roots of diseases materials, and receive exclusive content on our app. We look forward to joining you in your walk-out journey and being able to assist you. With God's help, we can do this together! To learn more, go to: beinhealth.com/partners.

For My Life®

For My Life is a one-week retreat hosted by Be in Health at our campus in Thomaston, Georgia. It is designed to help people who are seeking healing and restoration of their physical, emotional, and spiritual health. We believe that most diseases result from separation in relationship from God, ourselves, and others. This retreat will help you to identify and deal with the "root issues" that may be keeping you from being in health. The For My Life retreat consists of intensive teachings, group ministry sessions, time to interact with the teachers and ask questions, and a time for personal prayer for healing at the end of the week.

Be in Health endeavors to make For My Life a safe place for you to find hope and healing for your life. We also offer For My Life Online for those who cannot travel at this time. Go to beinhealth.com/for-my-life.

For My Life Kids and For My Life Youth

Every year in June and July, we offer For My Life for the whole family; that is the For My Life Adult, For My Life Youth (ages 13–17), and For My Life Kids (ages 6–12) Retreat all in the same week! This is an opportunity for the whole family to be transformed and healed from the inside out. We hear so many people say, "If only I had known this when I was younger, I would have been saved from so much torment and heartache!" We've listened and developed these specialized retreats to continue our mission of establishing generations of overcomers. In the For My Life family week, everybody in the family can benefit and be on the same page spiritually. We take the same information that is presented in the adult For My Life Retreat but reformat it to be relevant and engaging for each audience. Go to: beinhealth.com/for-my-life-kids-and-youth.

Be in Health Conferences Near You

Our Be in Health team travels too! We bring one- to three-day conferences to locations all over the world. If you want to find out more about these conferences and when one might be held in your area, or if you are interested in helping us bring a conference to your area, go to: beinhealth.com/conferences.

Social Media

You can also follow us on your favorite social media platform!
Facebook: @beinhealth
Instagram: @beinhealthofficial
YouTube: @BeInHealth
TikTok: @BeinHealth_Official

Other Books and Materials

If you enjoyed this book, you would love our other books and teaching resources in the Be in Health Bookstore. You will find an extensive selection of materials by Dr. Henry W. Wright, Pastor Donna Wright, and other leadership team members. Topics range from the possible spiritual roots of disease to how to overcome specific spiritual issues to teachings on sound biblical doctrine.

A More Excellent Way by Dr. Henry W. Wright

Our Identity by Dr. Henry W. Wright

Overcoming Allergies by Dr. Henry W. Wright

God Is Greater Than Cardiovascular Disease by Dr. Henry W. Wright

Real Solutions for Autoimmune Disease by Pastors John and Adrienne Shales

Insights Into Cancer by Dr. Henry W. Wright

Overcoming Depression by Dr. Henry W. Wright

Overcoming PTSD by Dr. Henry W. Wright

And much more!

ABOUT THE AUTHOR

Dr. Henry Wright believed that many human problems, particularly as they relate to health, are fundamentally spiritual with resulting psychological and biological manifestations. Because of his extensive research and insights into both the medical and spiritual aspects of disease, he developed a unique and fresh perspective on ministering to the sick. Through over thirty years of application, ministry, and personal experience, Dr. Wright discovered that many diseases have an often-overlooked spiritual root that must be identified and dealt with from a biblical perspective in order for true healing to occur. He successfully applied these principles in teaching and ministering to others, with astounding results, as God healed many people from their diseases, many of which were considered incurable.

Dr. Wright grew up knowing that God heals disease. Two months after his birth, his mother was dying of fibrosarcoma cancer with an aggressive tumor that had wrapped itself around her jugular vein. At church one Sunday, she repented of bitterness and cried out to God. Instantly, the tumor disappeared. One week later, her doctor was amazed to find no evidence of cancer in her body. No medical treatment had been administered. Consequentially, her healing broke a genetic pattern in her generations; her own mother had died of cancer soon after giving birth to her. She went on to live thirty-three more years! Her prayer was that her son would someday serve God too. Though she didn't see the fruit of that prayer in her lifetime, God was faithful to place a calling on Dr. Wright's life. Her healing set a standard within him against the enemy and against disease.

Dr. Wright held a doctorate in Christian Therapeutic Counseling from Chesapeake Bible College in Ridgeley, Maryland. He was the president and founder of Be in Health Global® and the senior pastor of Hope of the Generations Church in Thomaston, Georgia. Henry and his wife, Donna, faithfully taught and ministered to those who God sent to them. They also traveled all over the world, teaching in conferences and ministering about healing in Jesus's name. Over time, they established the impactful For My Life retreat in Thomaston, as well as other retreats. These retreats have brought tens of thousands of people to restoration and healing in God as they discovered the spiritual roots of disease and applied scriptural truths to their whole lives—spirit, soul, and body.

Dr. Wright's first book, *A More Excellent Way* is a bestseller in the Christian market, has been translated into seven languages, and has sold hundreds of thousands of copies worldwide. It has helped thousands of people recover from the devastation of disease and find healing in God's plan. His book *Exposing the Spiritual Roots of Disease* also provides biblical truths to those seeking answers for disease.

Dr. Henry Wright passed away on November 18, 2019. Because of his passion for the Be in Health ministry to accomplish the Father's will for generations to come, Dr. Wright, his ministry team, and the board of directors had already established plans for the future. Dr. Wright's vision and ministry continue under the leadership of Pastors Scott and Sarah Harper, son-in-law and daughter of the Wrights, as senior pastors of Hope of the Generations Church (HGC). Pastor Scott also serves as the CEO of Be in Health. Pastor Donna Wright, Dr. Henry's wife and co-founder of HGC and Be in Health, is actively involved with both the church and the ministry. Along with the other pastors and the elders of HGC, she continues to invest her life into carrying forth the vision of her husband.

Today, thousands of people are still welcomed to the Be in Health campus each year and to conferences around the country as Dr. Wright's legacy continues to bring healing and restoration to the people who God sends to them.

STUDY GUIDE ANSWER KEY

Chapter One

1. reason for; we don't know the reason
2. disease management
3. disease prevention and eradication
4. to forgive all our iniquities and heal all our diseases
5. a spirit, a soul, a body
6. sanctify it
7. 80 percent; separation on three levels
8. Separation from Father God—from His person, His love, and His Word; separation from yourself; separation from others.
9. reconciliation and restoration of relationship
10. People feel closer to Jesus because He is their Savior. Father God may seem much farther away in heaven, or He may seem like a "taskmaster" waiting for them to make a mistake.
11. We believe that God loves us because God is love.
12. the failure of an earthly father
13. to make us His son or daughter; came to us from our heavenly Father; we have been adopted into God's family; "Abba Father," which means "Daddy"!
14. believe; loves us
15. told they have no value by loved ones or thoughts in their head; believe they are junk
16. junk; love
17. We must set down those lies and repent to Father God of having believed them. Believe the truth instead.

18. by becoming bitter through injury done to us

19. defiles us and others, making us susceptible to disease

20. *"If we confess our sins, he is faithful and just to forgive us our sins, and to cleanse us from all unrighteousness."*

21. from Satan, not from God

22. the Accuser

23. Satan changes the Word of God.

24. Their eyes were opened; evil flooded in; they felt fear, shame, and guilt.

25. God knew it was Satan who had interfered with His perfect creation with the sole aim of bringing destruction. He wanted Adam to recognize it as well.

26. He defeated Satan by quoting the truth of the Word.

27. is a happenstance or accident; the villain, Satan, and his kingdom

28. *"For we wrestle not against flesh and blood, but against principalities, against powers, against the rulers of the darkness of this world, against spiritual wickedness in high places."*

29. principalities, powers, the rulers of the darkness of this world, and spiritual wickedness in high places

30. to form us into his image; the image of death

31. spiritual training; discernment according to Scripture; *"My people are destroyed for lack of knowledge."*

32. to the truth of God's Word; *"Bless the Lord, O my soul, and forget not all his benefits: who forgiveth all thine iniquities; who healeth all thy diseases."*

33. assessing faith in our lives; repentance of dead works; faith

34. A divine influence upon the heart, and its reflection in the life.

35. No, it's for Christians too.

36. bitterness, accusation, envy and jealousy, fear, anxiety and stress, anger and hostility, rejection, shame, unloving spirits, self-hate, occultism, and addictions

Chapter Two

1. blessings and curses, health and disease; *"I have set before you life and death, blessing and cursing: therefore choose life, that both thou and thy seed may live."*

2. blessed in the city and in the field, blessed in the fruit of their bodies and in the fruit of their planting, blessed with the good treasure of rain, blessed as the head and not the tail, called God's holy people

3. Look up Deuteronomy 28:15–67 and list some of the curses related to disease.

4. causal connection; cause and effect

5. It is conditional and serves as a warning for believers.

6. Because of the mercy of God. He offers a place to change course so that curses do not come upon you.

7. the result of a curse; hemorrhoids, insanity, anxiety disorders, torment, autoimmune disorders, depression, incurable diseases

8. This thorn is known as a "messenger of Satan." God was making provision for Paul to overcome it. (See 2 Corinthians 12:9.)

9. No, God doesn't bring evil upon us; *"Let no man say when he is tempted, I am tempted of God: for God cannot be tempted with evil, neither tempteth he any man."*

10. each person, their family, and their generations have a different weakness that can lead to sin

11. *vilification*; vilification; *villain*

12. Satan; villain in our lives

13. *Abatement* means "lessening" or "reduction"; Satan comes to abate, reduce, or take away the strength of our blessings from God.

14. A curse without a reason for being there cannot affect us

15. Yes, it did.

16. by continuing in sin

17. we give the villain who is behind that curse permission to wreak havoc in our lives; by disobeying God and His Word and obeying the law of sin instead

18. the law of God and the law of sin.

19. *"another law in my members; bringing me into captivity to the law of sin which is in my members"*; still happens in us today

20. goodness, love, justice, forgiveness, faithfulness

21. rebellion, lawlessness, falsehoods, hatred, murder, evil

22. Satan

23. to disease; *"Behold, thou art made whole: sin no more, lest a worse thing come unto thee."*

24. "you are healed" "your sins are forgiven"; our sins being forgiven and our bodies being healed have a cause-and-effect relationship

25. divine influence upon the heart

26. The amount of time God gives us to figure out what He is saying to us through His Word and through His Spirit.

27. We can repent and turn away from it and allow our heavenly Father to renew us in grace and mercy.

Chapter Three

1. the elders of the church pray in faith and anoint with oil; *"...if he have committed sins, they shall be forgiven him."*

2. to convict "evil people" of sin to turn from their wicked ways; *"All have sinned and fall short of the glory of God."*

3. sin; getting rid of the sins that are at the root of the disease

4. others already had, and he knew what the Word said in 1 John 5:17; *"There is a sin unto death: I do not say that he shall pray for it. All unrighteousness is sin: and there is a sin not unto death."*

5. Healing can be blocked if the spiritual root issue that led to the deadly physical disease is not dealt with. Left unaddressed, the natural course of the disease will cause the person's death.

6. the law of sin

7. She called the unforgiveness "sin," asked the Father to forgive her for bitterness, and asked the woman she was bitter against for forgiveness.

8. *"But if ye forgive not men their trespasses, neither will your Father forgive your trespasses."*

9. She had to be obedient. She submitted to the Word. She became a doer of the Word. *"But be ye doers of the word, and not hearers only, deceiving your own selves."*

10. you are not a Christian or that you are an evil person; New Testament believers

11. communicate and repent

12. our salvation; our sanctification

13. A lifelong process for Christians whereby, through the glories and trials of life, and through our obedience to God, we learn to *"walk in newness of life."*

14. running away from the Bible; so we might be brought to repentance and freedom, not condemnation

15. We *"are changed into the same image from glory to glory, even as by the Spirit of the Lord"*; the progressive present tense; being changed into Christ's image is an ongoing process

16. We are still being sanctified in our spirits, souls, and bodies.

17. They should be renewed. *"Be not conformed to this world: but be ye transformed by the renewing of your mind"* (Romans 12:2).

18. Our sanctification: embrace His truth, repent of following any aspect of sin, and allow Him to transform us into His image.

19. Become an overcomer; face the challenges of life and defeat them, in Jesus's name.

20. We reflect His nature as part of our nature; of sanctification

21. It is possible we become a reflection of the enemy's kingdom.

22. We can choose to release the offense to Father God and forgive the individual. Or we can embrace the offense and choose to hold on to the hurt so that it becomes a wound.

23. after unforgiveness, then resentment, retaliation, anger/wrath, hatred, violence, and finally murder or murder with the tongue

24. Produce disease in our body.

25. If a woman comes for healing from breast cancer in the right breast, her unforgiveness is toward a non-blood relative. If the cancer appears in a woman's left breast, it is related to unresolved bitterness in the woman with another female who is a blood relative.

26. tendency to respond to anger and stress with hopelessness and despair to the point of being shut down, marked inability to forgive, a tendency toward self-pity and self-introspection, a poor ability to develop and maintain meaningful long-term relationships without fear, a great tendency to hold resentment, poor self-image, the loss of a serious love object or the continued grief and unresolved issues relative to the love object, the loss of a significant life role, being fired or rejected in a vocational pursuit, loss of hope, hope deferred, denial about personal feelings and needs

27. a lack of hope and love in a person's life; shutting down; stuff their emotions inside and pretend the problems do not trouble them at all

28. entrust our life to Father God and release our hopes to Him; what we can see and what we can control

Chapter Four

1. For Christians, some of our thoughts are from the Holy Spirit; some of our thoughts are our own; other thoughts originate from Satan.

2. Because of the Holy Spirit, Christians can have the "mind of Christ." Unbelievers cannot receive the things of the Holy Spirit.

3. Through reading the Bible, realigning our thinking with God's Word, repenting of sin, and embracing God's ways and nature.

4. spirit with a soul and a body; the eternal part of you is a spirit

5. the enemy; spirit level; soul (mind) level; bring the roots of disease with them

6. Because Satan tempts us with a thought that sounds like it came from us, repeats that thought over and over, and deceives us into accepting it as our own.

7. I never do anything right. I am not really loved by anyone. I hate my life.

8. Satan uses those thoughts to control us spiritually, psychologically, and biologically; temptations

9. theta, alpha, beta

10. our waking functions related to our five physical senses; between our body and our soul or mind

11. a more relaxed, thoughtful, creative way of thinking; our soul

12. between our soul and our spirit; the Holy Spirit and evil spirits communicate with humans

13. theta brain waves; His nature and righteousness; also uses theta waves to train us in the law of sin

14. the biology of how our mind affects our body

15. through a biological event called protein synthesis

16. whether good or evil; a permanent part of your biology; your mind, your personality, and the way you think and act

17. temptations to bring on disorders and disease; dwell on His Word so we can live in health and freedom

18. our minds become overwhelmed with fear, anger, self-hatred, depression, hopelessness, and much more; no, Jesus cast out evil spirits

19. possessed; owned; cannot; vexed with, troubled by

20. *"For God hath not given us the spirit of fear; but of power, and of love, and of a sound mind"* (2 Timothy 1:7).

21. cannot tempt believers; physical body

22. the mind receiving lies and temptations from the enemy; actions in our body

23. are *not* our sin; *separation*; *separate* from who we are

24. by making sin and evil appear to be *one* with us; personality defects and tormenting thoughts

25. By recognizing that these thoughts are not our own but are from the enemy, by repenting of the sin of embracing these thoughts, and by having the evil spirits cast out of us.

26. renew our minds by building new pathways of thought in God's truth

27. No, it is not; the evil thoughts and follow after them; have to stay there

28. You must recognize what it is. You must take responsibility for what you recognize. Repent to God of participating in what you recognize. You must make what you recognize your enemy and renounce it. Get rid of it once and for all! When it tries to come back, resist it! Give God thanks for setting you free. Help someone else get free.

29. *"casting down imaginations, and every high thing that exalteth itself against the knowledge of God, and bringing into captivity every thought to the obedience of Christ"*; despite what we feel

Chapter Five

1. the ectoderm, the mesoderm, and the endoderm
2. brain, nervous system, cardiovascular system, heart rhythm, skin, hair, eyes, ears, and nose
3. fear; love
4. heart circulation, muscles, skeletal form, kidneys, bone marrow, blood vessels, lymph glands, and more
5. guilt; righteousness
6. liver, lungs, intestines, urinary tract, and endocrine system, which includes important glands such as the pituitary and hypothalamus glands
7. guilt; honor
8. the brain
9. the voluntary nervous system; allow body systems to function without thinking about it; your heart pumps, you breathe, and your digestive organs work
10. when your long-term memory from the enemy causes malfunction in your nervous system or any other body system so that they no longer work properly
11. the lack of *ease* or health within your spirit and your body's systems
12. your emotions and your memory; the amygdalae glands and the hypothalamus gland
13. the "fight-or-flight" reaction; storing your long-term memories; deeply experienced emotions, whether positive or negative
14. the hypothalamus; health and disease
15. the pituitary gland, the adrenal glands, and the hypothalamus gland; to secrete hormones that keep your body balanced and working smoothly
16. the hypothalamus
17. a healthy body balance of all the body systems; you will develop a disorder or disease
18. body temperature, thirst, appetite and weight control, emotions, sleep cycles, sex drive, childbirth, blood pressure and heart rate, production of digestive juices, balancing of body fluids
19. serious health problems occur
20. information, thought, language comprehension, problem solving; long-term memory
21. the amygdalae glands receive and interpret those strong negative thoughts as a threat
22. The limbic system kicks into survival mode, and the hypothalamus gland responds.
23. it may become overwhelmed, resulting in neurological misfiring, neurotransmitter imbalance
24. disrupted its proper function; serious destruction of your body and organs
25. gastrointestinal disease, sexual disorders, skin diseases (eczema, neurodermatitis, acne), diabetes, fatigue and lethargy, overeating, depression, insomnia, coronary artery disease, hypertension,

stroke, disturbances of heart rhythm, tension headaches, muscle contractions, backaches, rheumatoid arthritis, related inflammatory diseases, asthma, hay fever, immunosuppression, autoimmune disease

26. as the direct pathway to bring disease into our lives; the soul (the mind and emotions) is the bridge between the spirit world and the physical world

27. when we obey God's Word; he gets us to disobey God's Word, leading to imbalance, or dis-ease, in our bodies

28. unforgiveness, bitterness, self-hatred, greed, envy, jealousy, anger, hostility, fear, stress, and anxiety; they become a part of our long-term memory and a part of our biology; from the amygdalae to the hypothalamus gland, which triggers the wrong signals to other vital glands in our body; it can cause damage to our bodies and serious diseases

29. the hypothalamus; dis-ease of function, a full-blown disorder or disease

Chapter Six

1. peace; torment

2. It is a spirit of fear; as stress in our human minds and bodies

3. replaced the phrase *"spirit of fear"* with the word "timidity"; God; we may no longer recognize that it is the evil spirit of fear that tempts and controls us

4. the substance of things we do not hope for; they both project into the future, and they both demand to be fulfilled

5. "According to your *fear* be it unto you!"

6. Who you are deep within, and how you relate to God, yourself, and others, rather than primarily how your body responds to the natural environment around you.

7. a spirit of fear related to not feeling safe in love and relationships; fear and anxiety; avoid or push away relationships, become isolated

8. cortisol; to help us in fight-or-flight situations

9. an unchecked release of cortisol that goes drip, drip, drip like a leaky faucet; begin to weaken our immune system

10. No, cortisol destroys the immune system because of a spirit of fear.

11. consequences of cortisol

12. identify organisms that are dangerous to you and to destroy them

13. T cells serve as killer cells, attacking and destroying viruses and other invaders. B cells produce antibodies that also act like killer cells and destroy the invaders.

14. an antigen flag; the antigen flags of unhealthy invaders and attack and destroy them

15. are destroyed by cortisol; that attack natural substances such as grass, pollen, animals, perfumes, and certain foods

16. histamine; various "allergic" reactions, such as itchy eyes, runny nose, sinus headaches, and rashes

17. vitamins, herbs, and health food; because the source isn't nutritional, it's a spirit of fear; antihistamines

18. allow Father God to develop His nature in us; *"The fruit of the Spirit is love, joy, peace, longsuffering, gentleness, goodness, faith, meekness, temperance: against such there is no law."*

19. The mother cried out to God and repented for rejecting the child. Then she snuggled that baby boy and repented to him, asking him to forgive her, even though he couldn't understand.

20. Their fear of her allergic reactions to the environment had created an atmosphere of fear in their home and had blocked the child's healing.

21. A broken spirit or heart could dry up the soft tissue of the bone marrow, affect the white blood cells, and destroy the immune system.

22. She repented of bitterness that reminded her of painful hurts from the past and of fear that brought her into isolation, cast down thoughts of fear of loving and being loved, and chose to trust God's Word over fearful thoughts.

23. we feel the sting of abuse and sins against us; to tempt us to become wounded and bitter, taking in the offense against us

24. we become bitter and take those offenses inside us and dwell on them; be willing to forgive others, turn to Father God and ask Him to convict us of sin in our life, and focus on our relationship to the Father

25. Stand up in our family line, stop blaming others for our problems, and allow Father God to transform our life and provide a new path into the future for us and our generations.

26. give and receive love without fear; the pain they feel

27. fear; the truth of God's Word concerning the Father's love for us

28. our bodies will stop responding to the training of fear

29. Father God who loves us and repent for those spirits of fear

Chapter Seven

1. Yes, *"Thou shalt love thy neighbour as thyself"* (Leviticus 19:18; Matthew 22:39).

2. a difficult time forgiving other people; harshness toward others

3. the inability to give or receive love without fear; they are afraid and bound by a spirit of fear

4. self-hatred, self-accusation, self-rejection.

5. harbor grudges; it is not self-seeking

6. that Father God loves us

7. by standards of performance and accomplishment

8. with Father God; our Creator made us and sees us as valuable to Him

9. thoughts from Satan's kingdom that they don't measure up, and they are reminded of past failures that reinforce their negative image

10. and begins to misfire; and becomes compromised

11. The white corpuscles in the immune system mistakenly identify the antigen markers on the healthy cells in the body as a disease or an invader and attacks or destroys them.

12. attacking themselves spiritually in self-rejection, self-hatred, and self-bitterness; and the white corpuscles start attacking the body itself

13. the person believes they are the problem; that they are their own worst enemy

14. an unloving spirit that produces feelings of not being loved and not feeling accepted

15. with a spirit of fear (producing anxiety and stress) attached to it; rejecting who God's Word says you are and choosing to believe evil thoughts from the enemy instead

16. by making the decision to trust what Father God has said about us; that we are *"fearfully and wonderfully made"*

17. of an anti-Christ spirit

18. being bound by sin that will not let you accept God's righteousness for you; by exalting Satan's lies over the Word of God

19. accusations of others toward you, specifically authority figures such as grandparents, parents, teachers, and even peers; unmet expectations of acceptance and approval

20. Acknowledge it's an evil spirit, repent to the Father for embracing the expectations of others and for allowing this evil spirit to beat us up over failures, let go of these thoughts, and take hold of the forgiveness God has given us by faith.

21. a willingness to get back up and repent when he falls in life; *"For a just man falleth seven times, and riseth up again: but the wicked shall fall into mischief."*

22. from God alone

23. a hostile environment or unloving family environment, particularly with rejection from a father

24. an evil spirit of guilt; risen Christ and forgiveness

25. self-accusation; that they are not as good as everyone else

26.   a spirit of self-hatred; Why am I here? Who am I? Who cares?

27.   by realizing that the Father cares; accepting His love can defeat autoimmune disorders in your life

28.   a performance disorder driven by a spirit of fear and a spirit of self-conflict; extremely driven to do everything right to keep the people around them happy; burden bearer of others

29.   a performance disorder similar to the one causing Crohn's disease; the burdens of others, leading to self-accusation and guilt; decisions

30.   Psalm 139, especially verse 14 that you are "*fearfully and wonderfully made*" by Father God who loves you.

Chapter Eight

1. nutrition and exercise; self-control; the temple of the Holy Spirit

2. It is not because exercise is useless but because godliness is profitable both in this life and for eternity; righteousness

3. Make a choice to believe the Word of God and trust Father God as the One who ultimately sustains life.

4. Choose the verses to write out from Nehemiah 8:10, Proverbs 17:22, or Psalm 118:17.

5. there is no reason to keep living; omit the importance of living every day unto the Lord; you serve Father God, until you fly away

6. anger, rage, fear (producing anxiety and stress), hardness of heart

7. tempers explode, outbursts of screaming, throwing objects, striking out physically

8. tempting thoughts and feelings from Satan's kingdom enticing us to embrace the law of sin; high cholesterol and high blood pressure; compromise the immune system

9. more aggressive, ambitious, controlling, competitive, and impatient than other people; no

10. love, joy, peace, longsuffering, gentleness, goodness, faith, meekness, temperance

11. by looking to the Word of God and His ways to break away from the law of sin that has led to these addictive thoughts; whatever you set your affections on other than God

12. protection mechanism; they do not explode in anger; will sustain them

13. the forgiveness that has been extended toward us; a spirit of guilt telling us that we cannot be forgiven and a spirit of shame causing us to feel unworthy of God

14. *"Harden not your heart, as in the provocation, and as in the day of temptation in the wilderness."*

15. when a person doubts and argues with God and His Word. *"Take heed, brethren, lest there be in any of you an evil heart of unbelief, in departing from the living God."*

16. rebellion; teachable

17. to rule and reign in your heart; God is your answer

18. very troubled hearts; trust the Lord and rest in Him; *"Peace I leave with you, my peace I give unto you: not as the world giveth, give I unto you. Let not your heart be troubled, neither let it be afraid."*

19. will fail them because of fear; the future, one another, political outcomes, illness, and death; peace

20. the heart; you give him permission.

21. choose Father God instead, moment by moment; God's nature; Satan's nature

22. spirits of fear of tomorrow and projecting fear into the future; *"Take therefore no thought for the morrow: for the morrow shall take thought for the things of itself. Sufficient unto the day is the evil thereof."*

23. a spirit of fear which causes a human's heart to fail; they have to perform to make everything right

24.   a spirit of rejection with the manifestation of fear of man, fear of rejection, and rebellion; accepted, wanted, and loved

25.   a spirit of shame; fear of man, fear of rejection, and dread; nobody wants them, and they are unacceptable.

26.   spirits of anger and rage that reveal bitterness in a person's life; past offenses committed against them

27.   a spirit of self-hatred coming from a lack of proper love, leading to a spirit of fear causing insecurities and pride (which is false confidence); a lack of love and nurturing

28.   a spiritually hard heart; the spirits of doubt, unbelief, and rebellion; being corrected or told when they are wrong

29.   *"The Lord is merciful and gracious, slow to anger, and plenteous in mercy."*

Chapter Nine

1. consistently sad, anxious, empty, hopeless, helpless, worthless, guilty, irritable, ashamed, restless, lose interest in activities, have problems sleeping, concentrating and making decisions, withdraw into isolation

2. a chemical imbalance in the body; in the normal function of the brain's neurotransmitters of chemicals; mental illness and disorders

3. heredity, environmental issues, psychological elements, the side effects of certain medications

4. the influence of evil spirits, which are often the root cause of mental illness

5. the soul; getting rid of the evil spirits influencing the person's thoughts

6. spirits of self-accusation, self-introspection, and self-centeredness

7. being the origin of the sin that is tearing their life down; themselves and their negative thoughts, inhibiting their ability to place their faith and attention on Father God

8. shame; guilt; self-pity; the "superglue of hell" ; bringing it into the present

9. do not feel loved and accepted; regulating mood, thinking, sleep, appetite, and behavior

10. New Age; anything to come into your consciousness, leaving you wide-open to thoughts and temptations from an evil kingdom

11. Considering God's Word daily. *"I will meditate in thy precepts, and have respect unto thy ways."*

12. the things they don't want to think about; the enemy of a person's soul is still active in their life

13. Recognize the temptations of the enemy, face them, and defeat them through the power of His Holy Spirit and His Word.

14. taking personal responsibility for deciding which kingdom you will serve

15. grab hold of the truth of the Word of God and be an overcomer; the sanity of God's Word

16. Recognize feelings of hopelessness and despair do not come from God or yourself, repent of accepting these thoughts, renew your mind by God's Word, embrace forgiveness and freedom in Christ, cast down every imagination that raises itself up against the truth of God.

17. walk out their salvation and consistently renew their mind

18. to come out of isolation; they can help us bear our burden

19. Read Psalm 139, believe the Scriptures, trust in and actively apply them to your life; Word of God; decision to embrace it

20. feel accepted and are driven to find something to take the place of that lack of acceptance

21. through the Word of God and the love of God; will become stronger; will become weaker and weaker

22. fear; did not know how to love each other; abuse or extreme pressure to be perfect

23. love them with no strings attached; *"There is no fear in love; but perfect love casteth out fear: because fear hath torment."*

24. an enlarged amygdala as a result of a spirit of fear; because of the spirit of fear, they cannot process their surroundings or come to a proper conclusion

25. Come out of isolation, get back into fellowship with people who love them, and forgive the person who originally brought the fear and anxiety.

26. guilt and self-hatred; for past failures (guilt); a spirit of self-hatred

27. Repent of having a perfectionist mentality, believe in and receive the heavenly Father's love and forgiveness, and begin to trust Him.

28. self-loathing and depression; had any joy; under a burden of accusation from the enemy

Chapter Ten

1. he speaks in the first person; "I am so concerned about what will happen tomorrow."

2. because the mind is hounded by stressful thoughts and imaginations; giving and receiving

3. won't feel loved by other people as an adult; a spirit of fear

4. *"The fear of man bringeth a snare: but whoso putteth his trust in the Lord shall be safe"*; the fear of people; *"I will not fear what man shall do unto me"*

5. build and restore their fellowship with others; the church; learning to love one another

6. A malfunction where there is organic damage to the body—cells have been destroyed and organs have been damaged.

7. a dysfunction of a bodily system where no damage has been done to organs and no body parts have been physically destroyed; syndromes

8. anxiety, stress, and emotional trauma change the brain; align your spirit and soul with the Word of God; long-term memory

9. have been victimized; the lack of covering or nurturing; fear of abandonment; anxiety, stress, drivenness, and perfectionism

10. and cast their cares upon the Lord; taking on too many burdens

11. spirit of fear of rejection; drivenness to earn approval and love from an authority figure

12. to succeed for the wrong reasons; you have value; earn love; as our source of approval of success.

13. the person struggles with a fear of failing others; for their approval; in moderation is important

14. approval must come from God; *"There is no fear in love; but perfect love casteth out fear."*

15. involves a breach in relationship; If we feel a zing in our spirit every time we think of that person, then we know something is wrong in our heart.

16. a spirit of fear; physically or verbally abused by their father, experiencing a lack of love

17. the father; self-hatred in the father/husband; he will not be able to share the love of God with his family

18. It may be associated with our heavenly Father, causing us to remain separated from Him; repent of any bitterness and forgive the father who abused us

19. a spirit of fear; to cast down temptations to embrace the thoughts of fear for our life and fear of potential problems in our future

20. a spirit of rejection; they will be accepted by others; insecurity, fear of failure, fear of the future, and overall dread; a spirit of rejection

21. an *internal* conflict; an *external* conflict; opens the door for fear; is guilt over having the conflict and how they are handling it

22. to repent of the fear and self-rejection; their peace from God; trust Him with the relationship or issue

23. spirit of fear that projects real or imagined fears; release the situation to Father God; trust Him to bring answers

24. in the fear of man, such as peer pressure, and the fear of rejection; to trust Father God, believing His acceptance is all that we need

25. the fear of abandonment; He will never leave us nor forsake us

26. the fear of rejection, fear of man, fear of failure, and fear of abandonment; addictive characteristic; apply God's truth that they are loved in Him

27. Get rid of the root of sin.

28. self-pity; all tempted to embrace these fears; make all the difference in our lives

Chapter Eleven

1. cast down imaginations and fill ourselves with the Word of God in our thought life
2. It is important to walk out the process of our sanctification and stay on track with the biblical truths that set us free from disease.
3. follow up by defeating the lies of the enemy and embracing God's truth
4. *"Ye shall know the truth, and the truth shall make you free."*
5. the intellectually converted; by the Holy Spirit
6. having real faith based on the knowledge of a living God revealed in the Bible; on the cross by Jesus Christ
7. we meditate on His Word; *"But his delight is in the law of the Lord; and in his law doth he meditate day and night."*
8. but rather feed on it for some time; ponder it, pray about it, memorize it, and talk about it with God and with others; our long-term memory, a part of our personality
9. mindless meditation that opens the person up to evil thoughts and spirits
10. renewing our mind; *"I beseech you therefore, brethren, by the mercies of God, that ye present your bodies a living sacrifice, holy, acceptable unto God, which is your reasonable service. And be not conformed to this world: but be ye transformed by the renewing of your mind, that ye may prove what is that good, and acceptable, and perfect, will of God."*
11. cleansed from Satan's lies and thought patterns
12. evaluate our thoughts and compare them to how He thinks; confront bad thinking.
13. allows us to build new pathways of thought; we think, speak, and act
14. sanctification
15. the way that the world thinks and the way that it acts; delivered from the diseases that the world gets
16. They will remain captive to their thoughts and the disease.
17. Work out our own salvation in fear and trembling.
18. They become offended and do not follow through.
19. just to be a survivor; to be a thriver
20. debate, discourage, and drag us down; into the image of any other person; into the image of God
21. "But we all, with open face beholding as in a glass the glory of the Lord, are changed into the same image from glory to glory, even as by the Spirit of the Lord."
22. We can expect God to heal us from the diseases of the enemy because God honors His Word and His image.
23. recapturing and recovering what He lost; His image in mankind; power of the cross
24. into His marvelous light
25. the Spirit of God wants to set you and your loved ones free from disease.